HomeMade Muscle

HomeMade Muscle

All You Need is a Pull up Bar
(Motivational Bodyweight Workout Guide)

ANTHONY ARVANITAKIS

ISBN: 1512366404
ISBN 13: 9781512366402

www.homemademuscle.com

Warning / Disclaimer

THIS INFORMATION IN this book is presented with good intentions. You must though, consult your physician prior to starting any exercise or nutritional program, especially if you have any medical condition or injury that contraindicates physical activity. All forms of exercise pose some inherent risks. You must take full responsibility for your safety and know your limits. Some of the exercises in this book may be too strenuous or even dangerous for some people. Before practicing the exercises in this book, be sure that any kind of equipment or surface you train on is well maintained. Do not take risks beyond your level of experience, aptitude, training and fitness. If you are taking any medication, you must talk to your physician prior to using this e-book. If you experience any acute or chronic pain, consult a physician. This publication is intended for informational use only and I will not assume any liability or be held responsible for any form of injury resulting from the use of this information".

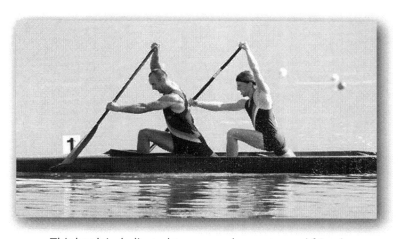

This book is dedicated to my coach, mentor and friend
Andreas Kiligaridis.
May he rest in peace...

Contents

Part 1

Losing a Leg & Becoming Whole

1

Hitting the ground

I T IS MARCH of 2008 and I am working the late night shift as a pizza delivery guy while finishing my studies in sports science and physical education at the Aristotelian University in Thessaloniki (Greece). I'm driving in a dark alley when suddenly big bright lights unexpectedly blind my eyes. I crash with a big automobile and I start floating through the air...

Movies tell you that in moments like these, time goes into slow motion and you see a reel of memories playing a short version of your life. Although I don't see a short trailer of my life, time indeed feels to be flowing a lot slower. What is probably a 3-4 second flight feels more like 15 seconds. I am experiencing a weird, but pleasant, state of weightlessness. It's s if I am going to keep ascending into the vastness of the dark sky.

Then suddenly, I hit the pavement, twenty-three meters away from the crashing point (as they inform me later on). I still haven't fully understood what happened. I try to get up and I look at my leg. Something is wrong. The lower part of my leg is twisted and my ankle... wait a moment that can't be right. I close and re-open my eyes to confirm what I had just seen. My leg is twisted in such a way that my ankle is lying on top of my knee. This is not a good sign, I think to myself.

The weird thing is that I feel no pain yet, which made me wonder if my eyes fooled me for a second. Fortunately, the human brain releases hormones that relieve pain in situations like these. Unfortunately, this doesn't last as long as you would want it to. Suddenly I sense a weird electrifying feeling. It is as if burning electricity is starting to flow through my leg. The endorphins that were relieving my pain start to fade away and the affected nerves start to wake up.

As I lay on my back, pain and fear start to overwhelm me. I hear people around me shouting to call an ambulance. With the side of my eye I can see a puddle of blood next to my leg on the pavement. I can't see much more than that because I am wearing long blue-jeans. I lay there and look at the dark sky while I feel people gather around me. The pain is growing stronger and stronger so I can't pay too much attention to them. I just close my eyes and hope that the ambulance will come as soon as possible to take me to the hospital (and hopefully numb the pain). At one moment I feel a presence next to me, I hear a male voice talking to me, trying to comfort me. I don't remember what he said but he gave me his hand and told me to squeeze it. I did and it helped a little bit with the pain.

After about twenty minutes, which felt more like hours, the ambulance finally arrives. They start placing me on the stretcher and the moment they lift my leg I start screaming. They pain is excruciating. We are now heading to the hospital and I'm in the back of the ambulance with a paramedic. He asks me if I have a phone on me and someone I should notify. I say yes and I reach into my pouch (you know the one pizza delivery guys wear). As I'm reaching for my phone I notice that the floor is covered with my blood. I have never seen so much blood in my life before so I start stressing out again. I asked the paramedic why is there so much blood? I haven't realized yet, that both bones of my lower leg, the tibia (the thick one) and the fibula (the thin one) are sticking out of my skin. So I asked the paramedic what is wrong with me, why is there so much blood?! I don't know why, but he doesn't respond. I asked again. "Hey man! Why is there so much blood, am I dying or something?" He doesn't answer again... "Well, that can't be a good sign" I think to myself.

I wondered for quite some time after my accident why he didn't answer me, or at least try to console me. Who knows, maybe it was his first day on the job and he was also freaking out. Anyway, back to the story.

The drive to the hospital seems like it takes forever. Because there are no available hospitals nearby, we had to drive all the way to the other side of town, which took a good twenty minutes. Twenty whole minutes on a bumpy road, and every bump firing up the nerves in my leg, causing me to clench my teeth and breathe heavily out of my nose. The paramedic reminded me to call someone, so I decided to call my parents. I took two deep breaths, and used a fake calm voice to inform them that I had a "little" accident and they probably should come to the hospital. When I arrive at the hospital I start to doze off as the pain is a bit more bearable. Maybe they have given me something for the pain, I don't know. Everything is really fuzzy, as if I'm in a dream.

Suddenly they take me in a room to clean my leg wound. I'm not sure but I think they are using some type of water hose, designed for these kinds of situations. The pressure of the water on the open wound brings me back into reality. This is probably the most uncomfortable sensation I have ever had. I start to groan again and the nurse tells me "relax its just water." Yeah right, I thought to myself; easy for you to say, you didn't snap your leg in two an hour ago. I am informed I have an open fracture and I'm going to be operated on the moment a surgery room is available. After that, I dose off again. I wake up in a surgery room and a surgeon with a very calm voice and a smile on his face starts talking to me. He asks me typical stuff like what's my name, where did I grow up and other similar questions to calm me down. But suddenly, the seriousness of my injury overwhelms me with horrific thoughts. I begin to think "what if I might not be able to run again?" I loved mountain running, especially on the cold and crisp-air highlands west of Greece, where I grew up. The thought that I might not be able to do that again makes me panic. I tell him I want to run again and that he HAS to fix my leg. I grew up being an exercise-nut and having a healthy leg meant everything to me at that moment. I was 23 years old and I felt too young to become crippled. A sweet sense of drowsiness disrupts my stressful thoughts. The anesthesia has kicked in. I slowly fall asleep.

After what I was told was a 5½ hour-long surgery I wake up vomiting. There's a reason doctors don't allow you to eat for a day before surgery I guess. It felt as if I was already puking for a while before I even came to my senses. The doctor was relieved that I woke up. "You got us worrying there for a moment champ." They had some difficulty waking me up, I am told later.

2

Waking up

THE NEXT DAY I wake up in a typical hospital room to the smell of iodoform (you know, that usual sterilized hospital smell). I feel...ahh, how can I say this eloquently? I feel like crap. My leg hurts, my back hurts, everything hurts and feels achy. I basically feel as if I have fallen off some cliff; like the coyote from Road-Runner. It makes sense; I did fly twenty-three meters before landing on the pavement after all. A team of doctors who are performing morning rounds pass by and they tell me I am lucky I didn't sustain any other wounds (besides a leg split open in two). One of them tells me that being in such good shape as an athlete probably saved me from a couple of more fractures.

I have all kinds of IV tubes attached to my arms; an electrolyte IV to keep me hydrated, antibiotics for a leg infection (I later learn I have) and a blood transfusion to replenish the blood I have lost. Its day one and I am already running out of patience with these stupid, uncomfortable tubes. I generally don't like wearing excessive or re-strictive stuff. I can barely tolerate a watch on my wrist and I don't wear a coat unless it's minus degrees outside. During the next few days, I was given five of those blood bags in order to replenish the lost blood from all the surgeries and the accident. The doctor who performed my surgery, and is responsible for me, enters my hospital room. He tells me they did everything they could to save my leg. Although they have reattached it, they had to remove an inch of bone, some muscle tissue and skin in order to avoid further infec-tions. If the infection didn't calm down they would have to remove more bone and tissue off my leg in the following days.

Less than twenty-four hours have passed since my first surgery, when I am informed that I need to be operated on again. As my doctors feared, the infection has started to spread. The antibiotics haven't managed to keep it under control. They take me back to the surgery room, once again give me general anesthesia and remove more bone and soft tissue.

Over the next 5 weeks I have another 4 similar surgeries. After surgery number 4, I wake up and look at my leg realizing that some weird metallic system is attached to it. The doctors pass by and tell me that it's called an external fixator - its purpose is to keep the fractured bones aligned until they heal. They tell me that the pins screwed in my leg... wait what? I ask them "what do you mean screwed in my leg?" I realize that this weird metallic device is not just externally attached on my leg as I first thought. It is actually screwed in it.

I'm still fresh out of surgery and highly medicated so I can't re-ally feel a whole lot, but the thought of having this weird system screwed in my leg makes it look more like a medieval torture apparatus than a modern system for fracture treatment. I ask them again to explain to me what exactly this device is. They tell me that external fixators are used in severe open fractures in order to immobilize bones and allow them to heal. They consist of a number of pins and thick screws which go through your skin and bone, entering one side of the affected limb and coming out the other end. These pins and screws are secured together outside of the affected limb with clamps and rods constructing this whole metallic frame.

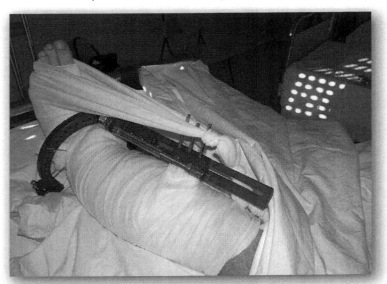

The medieval torturing apparatus I was telling you about...

The surgeries have worn me out, physically and mentally; I am tired and in constant pain. The pain treatment sucked. You see... Greek hospitals, mainly due to limited funding and corruption, are not the most ideal places to be hospitalized in the western "developed" world. Anyway, let's try and stay out of politics and let's focus on the story.

It's late at night and I am lying in bed unable to sleep. My leg pain starts getting worse and sweat is constantly dripping off of my back soaking up the bed. I press a button to call a nurse so I can maybe get some more pain medication. Half an hour passes and no response. I look at an old clock on the wall - its 3 a.m. I squint my eyes for a couple of seconds and when I open them its daylight. Nurses are passing by and family and friends are in the room. How can this be possible I think to myself, it was 3 a.m. seconds ago. I talk to the people around me but no one replies. My voice has a weird echo... I squint my eyes again and I'm back in the dark room lying on sweaty sheets. "Ok, relax" I say to myself. "You're just hallucinating from the fever and the drugs." Since day one I had a non-stop fever which made everything even worse. The doctors informed me that it was a normal reaction to the physical stress from all the surgeries, drugs and the open wound I sustained. Nightmares and weird hallucinations from the fever and drugs is how I spend most nights.

Another thing that makes these days seem endless is the fact that my back is also killing me. Your back can get extremely sore when you have been lying on it for days. At some point, my back hurt even more than my leg. One day I noticed a physiotherapist doing rounds with some students. You could see right through his fake attempts to impress the young female interns with that "I run shit here" attitude. I tell him my back is killing me and ask if he can do something about it. His response, "And why are you asking me about something like that?" I look at him with a dumbfounded look as he leaves the room. The only thing that comes to mind is the lyrics of my favorite rock poet, Jim Morrison "People are strange... ♪"

On week three, my doctor comes in with some bad news. He tells me that if the infection keeps on spreading they will have to amputate my leg. "We ought to inform you about this so that you can be prepared." I said, "ok" and pretended to be cool until he left the room, when I turned on my side and teared up a bit. I was tired and confused. How had my life suddenly taken such a turn? A week ago, I was sprinting along the seafront of Thessaloniki's Port at lightning speed and now I am in a hospital bed wondering if I'll have my leg sawed off. I am operated on again the next day and three days after that a team of doctors enters the room to update me about my situation. "You've dodged the bullet," they tell me. I feel relieved, for now...

Due to the trauma and all the surgeries to avoid infection, one-third of my lower leg had literally no skin. All that was separating it from thin air was the bandage that a medical intern would change every morning. In my last surgery, doctors took a skin graft from my thigh to cover the exposed part of my leg. In such situations like mine, skin-graft transplants are not the equivalent of cosmetic surgery. It's not like they cover the wound with what looks like normal skin. It's simply a thin layer of scar tissue that covers the wound and makes it look more like a third degree burn than anything else. To avoid infections, for the next couple of days an intern had to apply a form of acidic liquid on the wound and the healing skin. He had to do this every morning. Every day at exactly 11 a.m. he would enter the room and the torture would begin. You know that stinging feeling you get when you have a small cut on your finger and lemon juice comes in touch with it? Imagine the same feeling, and multiply it, let's say, about a hundred times. And there I thought my torture had ended.

3

Looking down

AFTER FIVE WEEKS in a hospital bed, five surgeries and countless feverish nights I have lost more than ten pounds. I also haven't walked for a month so my leg is extremely atrophied but I haven't really noticed yet. Because the lower part of the leg is swollen due to the trauma, I didn't notice how much muscle mass I had been gradually losing. Some nights I feel my abnormally thin thigh muscles when I rub them to divert the pain from the lower affected area of the leg. But when it's daylight I forget about it. Even thought I knew on some level that my thigh had lost a lot of it's muscle mass, I didn't expect to see what I saw when I observed my whole leg a week before I checked out of the hospital.

It's a Tuesday morning and my doctors tell me I'm going home in a few days. Once they leave the room I have a good look at my leg while as I'm trying to change my shorts. What I see shocks me. I look down and realize that my thigh is actually thinner then my knee.

How is this possible? I was in top condition a month ago. Sprinting on the beach, dead lifting in the gym, muscle striations and veins popping from my athletic legs... it now seems as if my left thigh belongs to someone dying of starvation. You see, our legs might have the strongest and biggest muscles in the whole body, but these muscles are also the ones that atrophy the fastest once you stop bearing weight on them. A few weeks of no walking were enough for what felt like maybe even 70% of my leg's muscle mass to disappear.

A nurse enters the room, "tomorrow you'll be allowed to stand up again," she tells me. "What do you mean," I ask, while feeling disoriented from my previous realization. "Well, you'll get started on learning how to move around with crutches on your healthy leg" she explains. I nod, open my laptop and put in a DVD with old Friends episodes a buddy of mine had brought earlier that day. I try to forget what I had just seen and maybe divert my attention enough to get a laugh or two. On the bright side, I had family and friends every day who also cheered me up a bit, or at least tried to... It's funny how in times like these people you think will be by your side vanish while others you least expect end up showing up every day.

Like my buddy Kostas for example. We had met 6 months ago, me being his Canoe Coach at the Nautical Club where I used to train and also work part-time during my studies. He was a hard worker and that's something I always appreciated as a coach in my athletes but also in people generally. We got along well but I didn't expect him to visit me every single day - for 5 whole weeks! He would try to cheer me up and also distract me from this whole mess I was in. Not too long ago, I was bossing him around the Nautical Club to do pull ups and work on his rowing technique but now our roles had switched. My doctors had me doing some toe extensions and flexions to keep the nerves in the leg active. I didn't really have the mood for it... So Kostas made sure I didn't slack off and motivated me to try even harder.

On the other hand, some lifelong friends didn't even appear. That's ok, I never kept hard feelings on account of that. I myself was a very different and shallow person back then, before all this.

I thought getting out of the bed would be easy. You see, until now due to all the surgeries, I wasn't even allowed to sit up straight on my bed. I was constantly laid on my back. A physiotherapist entered my room to get me started on some moving around with my crutches. I expected we would be doing that from day one. "So, am I going to walk today?" I asked. "Of course not," he tells me. "Day one is just about getting you to sit upright on the bed." The cocky ignorant voice in my head is going on saying "oh come on man, I'm not a hundred years old, I'm a strong guy for goodness 'sake."

The moment I stand upright on the bed, my heart starts racing, I start sweating and feeling dizzy. It was as if the moment I tried to stand up my body triggered an alarm. I laid down again wondering what is going on? Why is my body freaking out? They tell me that it's a common reaction in cases like mine. The body has been adjusted to being on a supine position for a long period of time and it overreacts when it has to compensate for the effect of gravity upon the change in the distribution of blood and blood pressure.

So, the next three days I just try to readjust my body in a standing upright position. It took three days to be able to do just that. Three days just to learn to sit straight up on a bed. Man how did I get to this point, I think to myself. After that, I slowly start walking on crutches. First walking three steps and back, then three meters and back, then to the bathroom and back, and after a week, I start walking a bit in the corridor outside my room. It was extremely tiring just to move around my bed; those walking attempts felt like the equivalent of an hour of mountain running. But they also started giving me a bit of confidence.

Forty-two days after my accident the doctors come in my room with, what is considered for them, good news. "You are going to be discharged in a couple of days," they tell me. I ask them, how long is my recovery going to take. "About a year," they reply. I'm startled..."a whole year?" I ask again. "Well yes, give or take. It will take a lot of time to re-lengthen your leg to cover the lost bone length, but we think we will succeed." You see the fixator they had installed on my leg (that medieval torturing device) besides stabilizing my leg's fractured bones, also had the ability to lengthen it.

The way this works is that every time your bones start to stick together, you turn a screw in the system that pulls the bones a bit apart until they re-build new bone tissue between the new gap and start sticking together. Think of it as teeth braces, but instead of aligning your teeth, it also lengthens them (bad analogy I guess, anyway). They told me that even short people who wanted to become models used external fixators to gain height. I think to myself - these people are definitely out of their mind to go through such torture just to become a model.

Once the doctors leave the room I try to digest the fact that I am going to be a patient for a whole year. It isn't easy, especially for a non-sedentary/exercise freak like me. How am I supposed to spend a year on crutches and sitting on my ass without going cuckoo?

4

The big depression

AFTER LEAVING THE hospital, I returned to my parent's home for my recovery. The thing I enjoy most of all during those first weeks is...eating! After six weeks of crappy hospital food and losing a lot of weight my body was constantly craving anything that has calories and a decent home-cooked taste.

The nights are still tough. I am constantly uncomfortable. Besides the screws and pins in my leg, the rest of my body also feels extremely restricted. After being a lifetime prone-sleeper my only option now is to sleep on a strict straight position on my back (due to the external fixator). I can't get used to it...I am constantly craving sleep but at the same time the leg pain and the awkward lying position I am restricted to prevents me from shutting my eyes long enough for Mr. Sandman to visit.

Any time I have to move, for example going to the kitchen to get a glass of water, I have to carefully walk on crutches - slower than a turtle. I also get dizzy most of the time I stand up so that adds extra difficulty to the task. I hate the fact that I need crutches for every little movement I have to do and wonder how handicapped people get through a whole life in this manner. My admiration for these people grows tremendously within a couple of days. People who spend a lifetime in wheelchairs and using crutches while maintaining a positive attitude deserve tremendous respect. They ground me and remind me that situations like mine are minor in comparison.

Still, I hated the condition I was in. For the next three months I didn't leave home. I had no desire to see or socialize with people. I just stayed in my room most of the day watching TV shows. Thank goodness we live in a golden age of TV and I have plenty of shows to distract my attention.

However, you can't watch TV shows all day on your laptop, you need a break at some point otherwise you get a headache. After those three months, I decide to start moving around a bit. A friend comes by and we go for a walk in the neighborhood. People stare at the metallic device screwed into my leg as if it is from outer space. Being an introverted person I hated the attention. I decide maybe it would be better to go out during the evening to attract less attention. The next day I had a routine check up with my doctor.

After taking some x-rays of my leg, I am in the waiting room with another dozen fracture related patients. A lot of them also have fixators on their arms and legs, which makes me feel as if we all share a silent comradery. It had been quite awhile since I was surrounded by people without feeling as if I was from another planet. Other than it's like any typical boring doctor visit. People in the waiting room looking indirectly at each other for what feels like forever. Others pretending to be reading something serious on their phone or flicking through some magazine pages. A couple of heavy sighs from patients who were in pain (some probably more dramatic and frequent than required). The buzz of the x-ray machine in the background and finally... hearing the receptionist call your name. I go in, say hello with a fake smile and give my doctor my x-rays. After looking at them with his team, he tells me, "we have progress." The bone seems to be healing and considering my youthful age and healthy background I probably won't have any problems with my recovery. After the appointment and for the next couple of weeks I gradually start feeling optimistic. Unfortunately this does not last that long.

A month later, and five months in total after my accident, the healing process has come to a halt. We schedule a new surgery. They have to install a different fixator in my leg and draw bone marrow from my pelvis and inject it in the fracture site. They explain this is a typical process performed to assist bone healing in extreme fractures like mine so I agree to go on with it. I thought I was done with surgeries so I wasn't thrilled when I heard I had to have a new one.

Unfortunately, the new fixator installed in my leg is now even bigger and more uncomfortable. The following months I suffer from extremely painful pin infections caused by this new fixator and I'm on and off heavy antibiotics and pain-killers all the time. Days, weeks and months keep on passing by. Winter, spring, summer...

trees grow green leaves, the leaves die again and I'm just waiting in my dark room, which is on the last floor/ attic of my parental home. Curtains closed, depressed and not in the mood for company. The leg continues to show no progress at all. On the right you can see the new, bigger and more uncomfortable fixator.

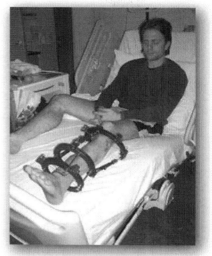

My doctors recommend a new surgery again. They now plan to remove a small piece of bone from my pelvis and place it on top of the fracture inside my leg. They explain to me this is another approach used in cases like mine and most of the time is successful. Man, I think to myself, what is next, leg transplantation?! They inform me that the down side of this procedure is that there might be permanent nerve damage on the side of my pelvis and the post-surgery recovery period is considered quite painful (which is the technical term for "it will hurt like a mother-f#$%r). A couple of hours after waking up from surgery, the anesthetic starts to wear off. I feel as if a horse has kicked me below the rib cage.

A couple of days later I am once again checked out the hospital and back to my attic room - or what I also had started calling that period "The bat-cave." Every time I had a check up with my doctor, I just asked how much longer... He always gave me the same answer,

"A couple of months more, have patience..." That was probably the worst part of all these years. Building hope every couple of months just to receive bitter disappointment again. The X-rays (which by now I have become an expert in examining by myself) only show a black disheartening gap. No white color, no calcium formations... just a black gap, which also resembled my mental state. I started spending most days in my room contemplating if an amputation would be a better solution. Whenever I talk about it with my doctors they tell me to have some more patience and not to rush into extreme decisions. Not to rush? It's been almost two years and still no results, what do you mean not to rush? I don't want to spend all my youth sitting in a dark room and having surgeries every couple of months!

Those were the darkest times of my life. Locked in my room, unwilling to do anything productive, feeling too tired to feel angry, feeling down. I have never felt so tired in my life before, even though I did nothing but sit or lay on my bed all day. Where is all this fatigue coming from I wondered. I had been an athlete most of my life, training for national championships, lifting weights, swimming 3km's, running up to two hours some days and training a total of 3-5 hours most days. Yet, I never felt as tired as I felt now. Just going to the bathroom felt like a whole journey. Physically, I felt as if I had grown forty years over the past twenty months. I guess depression does that to you.

Since I was young, I always had a tendency to get depressed and melancholic due to my nihilistic philosophy about life (Nietzsche was sort of my role model). But, exercise was a great way to distract me from those moods. Now, however, I was going through all this and had nothing to distract me from such feelings. My body felt heavy, my mind was constantly blurry with no energy to focus on anything. I would try reading a book, but after trying to focus on a couple of lines, my mind just became foggy and I felt worn out. I felt disconnected from everything and everyone. There would be days when I would spend all day in bed with some music playing in the background from my laptop speakers while I just starred at the empty ceiling. Those two years felt literally like an eternity. Some days I almost counted every single minute.

Everything was failing and my doctors once again proposed a new operation. They would remove a piece of muscle from my back and place it on top of the fracture where the skin quality was bad. "Because a lot of muscle and skin tissue has been removed in the first surgeries, the fracture-sight might benefit from some additional healthy soft tissue," they tell me. "Yet it's quite a risk because you are left with only one functional artery for blood supply in this area," they explain to me. I begin to think they must be making a bad joke.. When I understand they are serious about removing part of a muscle from my back and placing it on my leg, I decide I have had enough of all this and that I am going somewhere else for a second opinion.

After what had been two and a half years and a total of 8 surgeries and no actual progress in the last year, I decided to fly over to the Netherlands. I am also half Dutch from my mother's side and have a few folks there. The Netherlands have a good reputation in trauma medicine so I decide it's a good place to get a second opinion. I move to the Netherlands, find a good surgical team and get started with treatment again. After a couple of surgeries and two different fixators installed in my leg, the bone seems to start to healing again. A year passes by and they install an inner titanium plate removing my fixator. I'm finally fixator-free for the first time in three and a half years! You can't imagine what a relief it is not to have any metallic objects going through my leg after such a long time. Although I do have an inner titanium plate, I don't really care. I can't feel it that much anyways. I could finally sleep in a different position other than my back and walk outside without people staring at my leg as if it has some kind of alien technology installed on it.

After two months I have an inner infection again and they are forced to remove the plate. Still the bone has healed quite a bit and they tell me that it might completely heal in the following months even with just a leg cast. After three months my doctors allow me to walk again and I start rehabilitation. Something, though, doesn't feel right. It is as if my leg will crack and break if I put too much pressure on it. It just doesn't feel sturdy enough. I inform my doctors and we do some x-rays, but nothing really shows up. It's probably normal to feel like this after not walking for so many years; apparently it's just psychological I think to myself. Until, one day I trip while crossing the road and the bone breaks again. There I was, after four and a half years of walking on crutches and canes, having six different metallic systems screwed into my leg and severe depression - back to square one. Waiting on the side of the road for my second ambulance ride. This must be big long nightmare I think to myself. Maybe I was left in a coma after my accident and I'm just imagining all this.

A couple of days later, I am once again lying down on a couch at home with a broken leg, staring at the wall. They had put a splint on it, hoping it would heal. Since the skin of my leg was so destroyed from the accident and all the prior operations, it couldn't sustain any more surgeries. Two months pass by and the bone-healing rate is minimal.

5

Ending a Five Year Odyssey

THE DOCTOR'S SOLUTION to my desperation was as usual, "have more patience." That summer my mental health had regressed. Out of the blue, I started having panic attacks. My heart would race and the air in the room felt so dense as if I had to swallow it to breath. My hands would suffer from extreme eczema breakouts. They would suddenly get covered with painful red blisters, to the point where I couldn't even use my crutches. So there I was, me and my useless, deformed limb that didn't even look like a leg to me anymore. Not able to even use my crutches to go to the bathroom and struggling to breathe.

Until one day, I said to myself I had enough....

I decided to chop off what was left of that useless part of a leg I was dragging around for the last 4 years and I would go on with my life. I told my doctors I wanted to amputate (feeling like a fool that I hadn't done this earlier). Even though none of my doctors had recommended it until now, I knew that it was the only true solution. The doctors respected my opinion and finally told me it was a better choice if I wanted to have an athletic lifestyle again. After making this huge decision that day and after receiving my doctor's approval, I felt liberated. It was as if a huge weight I had been carrying with me all those years since my accident, was lifted. After a lot of time I felt a sprinkle of self-confidence again.

That summer was a huge revolution in my life. I would wake up every day feeling like a different person. I believe that people rarely change, but a life tragedy can offer the proper conditions for this to happen. After being depressed for four and a half years, I decided I was just tired of feeling like crap. I wanted to be happy again. Within a couple of weeks I was transformed. Meditation played a huge role in all this and it was what got 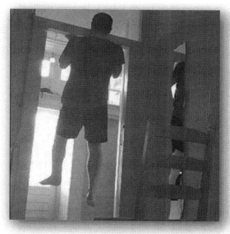 me started on my journey of self-improvement. I don't remember why, but I ordered a book about meditation I had found online. It was written by a Tibetan monk and a science reporter for the New York Times. The book talked about how meditation had been proven to have positive effects on the brain and other cool stuff like that. I thought why not give this a try. After starting to meditate I also decide to feed my body with proper food and to start some strength training.

Although I need crutches to move around, and going to a gym isn't an option, I am determined to find a way to workout. So I start developing a home bodyweight routine. I just did a couple of pull ups, push ups, leg raises and dips in the beginning. I don't have any equipment so I used a door-frame to do my pull ups on (picture below) and a narrow stairway to do my dips. Even though this wasn't a lot, my muscles started to wake up again. As body-fat started to fall off, muscular curves and vascularity began to emerge beneath my skin. My reflection on the mirror started to remind me of my good old fit self - it was really empowering. My hand eczema started to subside and my brain-fog started to clear up, so I started reading more books. I became obsessed with anything I could find on health, nutrition and exercise but also on self-improvement.

The surgery was scheduled in six months and I promised myself that I would be prepared for it in every possible way. As an athlete most of my life, having a strong body was something that also supported me mentally. I don't know about you but when I'm in good shape I feel more rooted to the ground. My body and mind feel sturdier. So, I knew that if I wanted to face this surgery with courage and tenacity, I would have to be strong both mentally and physically. For six months I trained consistently both body & mind. Meditating, strengthening my muscles and eating healthy. It all paid off. I was feeling healthier than ever and my body was in great shape. I was ready to face the big challenge.

The big day

It's January 17th and Amsterdam is covered in snow. I am looking out a hospital room window at the snowy scenery. After waiting peacefully for a couple of hours a nurse enters and tells me with a soft smile that it's time. I'm reflecting to my situation and my own calmness amazes me for a brief moment. I never thought someone could be heading to surgery - to have his leg cut off, without experiencing severe anxiety, especially when this person was me. I had been extremely calm these past few months, mainly thanks to my new daily habit of meditation. However, a part of me was wondering if I would freak out the day of the big operation. My heart beat raised and my hands felt unsteady a few times. However, a couple of seconds focusing on my meditational techniques were enough to remove the tension. I simply reminded myself that this all was for the best and observed my physiology's response to my emotions until they melted away.

As I lay on the surgical table I say to myself - this is it. My palms feel shaky again as I realize that a part of my body which I have been carrying around all my life will disappear. But, my mind is at peace. I accept that this is a huge turning point in my life and that it's only going to be uphill from now on. The anesthetic slowly starts to kick in and my vision becomes blurry. I can only see the gloomy white lights on the ceiling. Once again I enjoy the feeling of weightlessness and I let myself fall asleep.

A couple of hours later I wake up and a nurse tells me the surgery went well. I am freezing cold which is a typical post surgery reaction. The nurse brings me a heated blanket. Suddenly I realize I still feel my leg. Did they do the amputation? I ask. The nurse tells me yes. What's weird is that I still feel my leg, and even though I was prepared for this, the sensation was remarkably realistic... it's called phantom limb, and if you've never heard about it before, it's the sensation an amputee experiences when the amputated limb still feels attached to his body. Approximately 75% of amputees experience phantom sensations in their amputated limbs. Some of the typical sensations are pain, warmth, cold, itching, tightness, and tingling.

Luckily, I didn't experience that much pain, not even in the beginning. My main feelings where pressure and an extremely annoying itch which kept me sleepless for the first three weeks. Thankfully that also subsided. A week after, I was discharged from the hospital and had to rest at home for three weeks before any kind of rehabilitation could begin. However I didn't want to get completely out of shape and, being the stubborn person that I am, I started doing some pull ups after day 4 at home. I was also extremely eager to begin walking on my prosthesis. Rehab took 5 months and I was finally able to walk without crutches again. Once I started to walk, I woke up every day early in the morning and went for a stroll to practice my gait. I loved those mornings - the feeling of freedom was incredible. Walking with my chin up, no crutches, no canes and without the hunched-up depressed posture I had all those years was something that felt extremely empowering. It still does, maybe not as much as those days but whenever I need to uplift myself, going for a prideful walk always refuels my self-confidence.

6

Life Insights From Losing a Limb

ALEXANDER THE GREAT was once faced with a terrific challenge. In a city named Phrygia, there was a famous knot - called the Gordian knot. Nobody could undo this knot and the oracles foretold that the person who would accomplish this, would also rule Asia. When Alexander arrived in the city of Phrygia he spend some time trying to figure out which way the ropes were wrapped and attempted to find a smart way to untie the knot. As a lot of eager ambitious men had done before him, Alexander struggled, became frustrated and in the end failed to loosen it. He suddenly stepped back and called out, "what does it matter how I loosen it?" With that, he drew his sword, and in one powerful stroke, he severed the knot.

Sometimes the only way to move forward in life is by cutting off that piece of your past which you've been dragging on and on. Sometimes you just have to leave things behind. We all carry stuff from the past that are holding us back from what we really want to do. Either that's people, bad memories, negative mind-sets (conditioned through a lifetime growing up), a useless limb or as in my situation: all the above. Sure it's scary; it takes tremendous effort and a lot of courage. Being courageous though is not about being fearless. It's about accepting fear, looking deeply into its core and moving forward anyways. Melancholy and passive negativity are two of the mind's most favorite companionships. Getting rid of this two-headed monstrous state of mind requires audacity. Remaining depressed and motionless when life gets hard is easy. It does not require any effort, it's a state of mind that arises by itself and the more you stand still in it, the more it paralyzes you. The more it becomes a swamp of quicksand that keeps pulling you in.

When life has thrown you down on your knees, be courageous. Look fear in the eye and cut the Gordian knot that is holding you back. It's not going to be easy and most of the time it will take a lot more than one strike of the sword. You will have to fall and rise up a thousand times. But the goal is not to remain standing. The goal is to learn that if you can get up once you can do it again. You develop a sort of muscle memory in overcoming adversities and you learn to do this more efficiently every time. Don't look at life as a sprint, but a marathon. A marathon filled with challenging obstacles. Everybody goes through dark times and everybody has those moments when they lose faith. When you are going through hell though - simply keep on going, as Winston Churchill once said. Because once the darkness passes by and daylight slowly starts to appear, you always wake up stronger.

Just do the best you can within your circumstances and in the process, if possible, try inching forward in the world just a little bit. If you cannot do anything about your own situation, find others you can help and support. Helping others grow stronger is sometimes the best way to strengthen yourself. I guess this is part of what HomeMade Muscle is about...

The days we live in, compared with all historical times, are some of the most prosperous. If you're not born in what is considered a third world country then you are going to suffer a lot less disease, war and hunger than most humans have who lived on this planet.

However, even though we might not face as many external challenges, we definitely experience equally difficult internal challenges. Even though we're not confronted daily with dangers that threaten our lives, we do experience negative emotions almost every living hour. Even after all I went through with my accident, and even though I could go through a leg amputation with an extremely calm attitude, I still have days when the tiniest things stress me out. Why is that? Well, the first simple reason is that life is unexpected. We don't always have the luxury of knowing when a demanding situation (like amputation surgery) will happen. We don't always have 6 months to prepare for it in the best possible manner. Shit just happens - unexpectedly! And because we are human we react emotionally. We become angry, scared, anxiety gets the best of us and we might even do the worst things to the people we love the most.

We can thank and blame our human biology for that because it's how a part of our brains are wired in order for us to survive. We evolved from an environment very different from the one we currently inhabit. As a result, we carry all kinds of biological baggage.

Our brains convert daily situations into potentially harmful threats. For example, when we're angry, blood flows to the hands. This makes it easier to grasp a weapon or punch a potential enemy. Heart rate increases, and a rush of catecholamine hormones such as adrenaline produce a burst of energy to face this threat. When we experience fear, blood goes to the large skeletal muscles, such as in the legs. This makes it easier to run away from predators that might be hunting us. It's also what makes our face turn white as blood is shunted away from it (creating the feeling that the blood runs cold).

Now here is the good news. We are also not the limited anxious organisms we once thought we were. Advances in science have shown that the brain has great flexibility in changing the way it is wired - what is also called Neuroplasticity. As Mingyur Rinpoche says in his great book, The Joy Of Living, "most people simply mistake the habitually formed, neuronally constructed image of themselves for who and what they really are." A great way to change these negative thinking patterns and images is meditation. When we meditate we adopt the objective perspective of a scientist toward our own subjective experience. Practicing meditation can help us develop daily awareness. This awareness can help us see things more clearly.

For example when our cup of coffee spills all over our freshly washed clothes, we can be aware of how minor of a problem this is, smile and change our shirt instead of going crazy over it. Instead of starting to curse, yell and waste the rest of the day feeling angry over a simple cup of java, we can take a step back, look at the situation as an external observer and just laugh. We can build positive reactive skills like these, and later on implement them into even more serious situations. Sadly though, for most of us, minor things like beverage accidents become levers for negative emotions which trigger patterns of negative reactions and behaviors (anger, disappointment, etc) that continue throughout the rest of the day or even more.

Surely, we are not always capable of reacting calmly. No matter how well you train yourself, your emotions will sometimes get the best of you. However, instead of soaking in an emotional lake of anger and stress or what is considered your "flight or fight mode" there are other alternatives to consider. You can find ways to discharge. Daniel Goleman, in his book Emotional Intelligence says, "All emotions are impulses to act." They are the instant plans for handling life that evolution has instilled in us.

Therefore, discharging negative emotions with some physical activity is a great alternative. When you are overwhelmed with fear in life, go for a power walk or a run to move all that blood flooded in your legs. When anger is controlling you, do some strength training. Once you're done, sit down quietly and observe the world around you. Realize that you're the one making everything much more dramatic than it is.

Look around you and usually all you'll see is stillness. People doing their thing, not even caring about you. Even if hostile people are surrounding you, observe their irrational behavior for what it is: impulsive, emotional reactions caused by problematic biological baggage. You might not always be able to control your exterior environment but you can always control your reaction to it. That's all meditation is for me...just shutting off the crazy emotional side of the brain and observing reality through an unbiased relaxed lens. You simply sit inside the eye of the cyclone and leave the rest of the crazy world spinning around you. If you don't keep on feeding anger, fear or sadness with more anger, fear or sadness, you can't really remain in such a state for too long.

Now take deep breath and observe the calmness around you. Rest that drama-queen lizard brain inhabiting your skull and slowly observe how much suffering you can save yourself by implementing this mindset in your daily life.

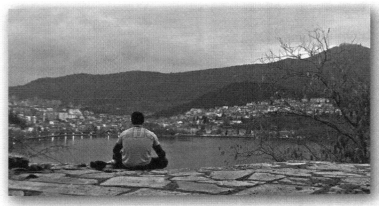

Kastoria - My beautiful hometown back in Greece

Part 2

Master the Basics

I LOVE EXERCISE; strength training, fitness, physique enhancement, running, swimming, rowing, you name it. It has been a part of my life ever since I took training seriously by joining my hometown rowing team at the age of 12. Since then, committing to the disciplined lifestyle of an athlete has equipped me with many helpful skills to deal with life's challenges. Leaving the world of professional sports caused me a great deal of disappointment due to not accomplishing as much as I aspired to. Fortunately I can now see the bigger picture in life. I can see how exercise can be a friend in lonely times, a place where I can find comfort and peace or a medium I can funnel my fears in and express my anger through.

Having purchased this book, I am hoping you also have at least some interest in health and exercise. If not, then at the very least, I hope my story intrigues you into developing a relationship with strength exercise and healthy habits as we go ;)

Ever since I began this project I have been faithful to bodyweight exercise. Whether I train at home or outside at a park, I always use bodyweight exercises. This way I stay loyal to this project and serve you - the people interested in home workouts - in the best possible way. I consider myself a lifelong student, constantly studying and learning the latest developments in athletic nutrition, strength science and bodyweight exercise. I am constantly keeping my mind busy on how to implement this knowledge into my project. I want to ask you to give me the honor of trusting me as your trainer. At least for a while to help you get started. By purchasing this book, you have in a sense, hired me to show you the best way to become strong and lean without going to the gym. When I commit to someone I always do my best to help them reach their goals. This is my duty as your trainer.

Keep in mind that because of this, I might occasionally disrespect what you consider traditional exercise information and I might challenge some of your ideas on exercise and nutrition. In this book you will read things such as "breakfast not being the most important meal of the day" or that "you don't have to do any more than 15 repetitions if your goal is fat loss." These sorts of things might be old news to some people like fitness enthusiasts who stay in touch with the latest developments in exercise and nutrition. But, because we live in an age of misinformation they might be new or even considered irrational for others. For the latter, I simply ask you to keep an open mind to what I have to say, examine the science behind these ideas and give them a fair chance before rejecting them. A lot of the myths I will be dispelling, will be myths I also suffered from until I started using an evidence based approach to exercise and nutrition. If you have spent the last several years reading the wrong exercise blogs, books and fitness magazines, it might be difficult at first.

Zen story

Nan-in, an ancient Japanese Master once received a very educated person who came to inquire about Zen. Nan-in served tea. He poured his visitor's cup full, and then kept on pouring. The guest watched the overflow until he no longer could restrain himself. "It is overfull. No more will go in! "Like this cup, Nan-in said, "you are full of your own opinions and speculations. How can I show you Zen unless you first empty your cup?" Try to empty your cup for the following six months and give this program an honest try. If you are a total beginner in strength exercise and your cup is almost empty, even better!

1

Who Should you Trust?

ON MEYER, A famous basketball coach, once said: "It is always easy to do right, when you know ahead of time what you stand for." I love this quote and this is why I considered it important to write this chapter. Ever since I started Homemade Muscle, I try to keep it supported by the latest developments in exercise and nutritional science. I have the fortune of being surrounded by very intelligent people who help me stay up to date with everything. At the same time, I spend every day studying and also filtering everything through experimentation in my own laboratory - my body.

> "It is always easy to do right, when you know
> ahead of time what you stand for"

Personal Results Are Good But Not Enough

I have put hundreds of training hours in this project and my personal results show that I practice what I preach. Still, keep in mind that someone's personal results are not enough to put your faith on. You shouldn't trust someone who uses solemnly personal experience to back up his opinions. There are numerous people in the fitness community who do this and the information they spread is to some extent (if not to a great extent) wrong. Many of them just have amazing genetics or use illegal substances such as steroids. Unfortunately, this does not mean their information will apply to the average Joe. As shown in studies people using steroids can get better results than people who exercise, sometimes even if they don't exercise at all! Of course it's a good sign that the person you trust has an analogous image to what he is preaching. I am a bigger fan of people who practice what they preach and have the results to show for it. But, that alone, should not be a reason for you to put your faith in him. There are some incredible coaches out there who look like they don't even lift due to crappy genetics. This becomes their personal reason and motive to become so passionate about finding the best way to supplement their efforts through solid knowledge.

If you want to be a proper coach and trainer, personal experience cannot be your only reference point. The fitness world is a wild jungle filled with deception, self-proclaimed gurus with God complexes, pseudoscience and scam artists. For those of you who are fitness and health enthusiasts and want to avoid being victimized, as I've often been in the past, I have included some guidelines that can help you avoid these pitfalls.

Science is Good But Not Perfect (yet)

Science is for sure the best place to start in this crazy world but... it is not perfect. When it comes to exercise and fitness, studies performed in universities have limitations. For example, when it comes to basics of strength training like ideal repetition ranges, or how many sets should an advanced trainee do; this area of research is hindered with difficulties in comparing studies. For example, the testing groups used are quite small, and in many cases they might even be undergraduate students who either are beginners in strength training or even subjects completely un-trained. Due to this, the "newbie gains" effect can interfere with the study, producing biased results. The newbie gains effect is the phenomenon of adding muscle and strength in a faster rate when you are a beginner in strength related training. This also happens, to a great extent, regardless of how optimum the train-ing program that is being utilized. In addition, men around the age of 18 might still be developing and therefore their hormonal profile will be a lot more optimum for muscle growth than some-one in his forties.

On the upside, we live in a great time for exercise science. Breakthrough studies are being performed on topics (such as the recent study on 'Recommendations for Natural Bodybuilding") by great people like Brad Schoenfeld & Alan Aragon who are some of the people leading the movement towards evidence-based in-formation in nutrition and exercise science nowadays. Research is gradually starting to focus more on trained populations. The more of these studies accumulate, the more of a solid ground there is to make clearer conclusions. No doubt, these are very interesting times for evidence-based fitness. And even though there is not enough science based on bodyweight exercise, I will do my best to integrate these two (bodyweight exercise and weight-lifting science) in the best possible way.

Avoiding Fitness Deception

When you want to be sure that a health authority, organization, you-tuber or blog can be trusted, ask yourself the following questions:

1. Do they help you understand their approach or do they get emotional when being questioned?

Someone who has knowledge on a topic should also be able to teach it. It is also very important is hear people once in a while say, "I don't know." No-one knows everything and if someone is trying to give you that impression he is probably trying to fool you. Many times people ask me something and I simply answer, "I don't know." Even if I think I know the answer but I am not 100% sure, I've learned to acknowledge my lack of knowledge and experience rather than mislead someone with incorrect information.

2. Do they use their credentials instead of solid references to make heavy scientific claims?

Basing something on the fact someone has a Dr before his name or a PhD after it, is not a good enough reason to trust some-one. This is the common fitness-trap I fell into when I started this journey. Also, remember that references should be based on articles and studies published in reputable places (not Wikipedia).

3. Are they willing to admit they are wrong?

When health authorities are stuck in old outdated information and aren't capable of acknowledging failures or facts that have been disproved in their program, it's a clear indication that they are more concerned with preserving their image than actually helping people. Realizing that I have used outdated data or have made a mistake and instantly admitting it has been one of the best ways for me to learn. I'm fortunate to have a network of very smart people around me, so I can't get away with mistakes anyway.

4. Do they have financial and/or emotional motives behind of what they are promoting?

It's normal of course for a health/fitness professional to make money from his projects and work. I'm certainly not unhappy whenever I sell an eBook, because it gives me the chance to invest even more money in this project and improve it in anyway possible. Still, this should also be a reason to remain cautious. If someone, for example, is selling muscle gaining supplements on his website be cautious when he is making extreme claims such as "my program with the right supplements can help you build 20 pounds of muscle in a month."

Feel free to question what I say. It's the best way for you and me both to learn and expand. If I believe I have made a mistake in this book, I would gladly accept an email from you and discuss your concerns.

Quick Summary

In conclusion, the HomeMade Muscle code consists of a Bruce Lee-ian approach to exercise and nutrition but it's also filtered through science. Here are my four most important suggestions for you:

1. **Research and question everything.**
2. **Absorb only what is rewarding and focus on perfecting it; Reject the rest.**
3. **Once you're mature enough, give it a touch of your personal experience and needs.**
4. **Simplicity is key to brilliance (Bruce Lee Quote)**

I haven't really created anything new in this home workout program. I have just constructed a simplified hybrid approach to home-strength and fitness development infused with the best information of Nutrition, Bodybuilding, Strength Training and Calisthenics.

2

Strong & lean without going to the gym
Is it possible?

WHEN I FIRST started the HomeMade Muscle project there were days when I used to chat online or Skype with friends, telling them I just finished my home workout routine. Most of them thought I was just fooling around doing a couple of push ups and pull ups and didn't really take me too serious. A couple of months later, when they saw how my body started to change they were amazed. "All that, just by training at home with no equipment at all?"

Paralysis By Analysis (PBA)

Today I try to show people that it's not about complex workouts, secret training techniques that "shock your muscles" and diets that have you eating magic berries and drinking weird colored beverages. Paralysis By Analysis is a common paradox that plagues the fitness community and one of the main reasons we consider getting in shape so difficult. The internet is one of the mains reasons this paradox exists and if you were born after an internet connection was available in every household, you have an even bigger chance of suffering from this paradox. Do not worry, you can get rid of this problem now that you are using HomeMade Muscle. PBA is a common problem nowadays among people who are trying to get in shape (I've also gone through it). In order to give you a better picture of this conundrum, I'll share with you a story by Aesop, the great ancient Greek fabulist. If these stories bore you, just bear with me for a few more lines.

"A cat and a fox discuss how many tricks and dodges they have in order to avoid their enemies. The fox boasts that he has many; the cat confesses to having only one. Just at that moment, they hear the cry of a pack of hounds coming their way. The cat immediately scampered up a tree and hid herself in the boughs. The fox lost in confusion, unable to choose between the plethora of all its tricks gets killed..."

Develop The Cat Mindset

That is precisely the problem that most people face nowadays when they fail to get in shape. Most of them carry the fox mindset. They have all this abundance of free knowledge accumulated in their heads from surfing around the internet all day but they end up neurotic and unable to stick to a single exercise plan. I even see this happen quite often with exercise professionals. They have so much knowledge accumulated in the heads, yet for some reason they seem as if they are too afraid to apply any of it. They are afraid that it just might not be the perfect workout plan. As a result, they end up switching from program, to program, to program... My advice? Be a cat! Ok that might not sound that masculine, but think of big manly ripped cat like Liono from the Thunder Cats (if you are too young and don't know what a Thunder Cat is, you are missing one of the greatest cartoons of all times).

On the other hand that is why people in prisons get so jacked up. They have very few means of training to choose from and a very big motive to fuel them. It's about survival, you have no choice.

Conclusion
The basic reasons most of us fail to attain our fitness goals is that we do not appreciate simplicity. We prefer complex approaches and ideas wrapped with fancy and shinny material. We look for the easy way out in everything we want to accomplish. Why train hard four hours a week when Cindy the fitness chick (with that stunning bosom) tells you that you can get ripped by training 12 minutes a day. We want exercise apps on our phone as if we are not wasting enough time on our smartphones already...

Screw all the fancy marketing fitness hype! Focus on finding proper guidance, consistency, and eating right.

Underestimating Bodyweight Exercise
Bodyweight exercise is commonly underestimated. Have a look at gymnasts or the new viral trend that has arisen on YouTube the several last years. People all over the world are training with only bars

and bodyweight exercises, doing what they call Street-Workouts and Calisthenics. You can see incredibly amazing physiques on these guys and they're just training in their neighborhood park. How cool is that?

A recent study found that people's ability to get up from the floor with no support from their hands was an accurate predictor of fitness—and even mortality. I don't know about you, but avoiding early death would be one of my top motives for getting in shape and taking bodyweight exercises seriously. I don't care if you can curl ninety pounds; if you cannot do ten strict pull ups, chest to bar, I don't consider you strong.

Bodyweight exercise provides a sense of personal mastery, control and self-confidence. What can be more empowering in the physical realm than mastering your own body? That is one of the main reasons I believe bodyweight exercise is superior to barbells and machines; that is if one must choose between one of the two. The bodybuilder physique was the ultimate accepted status quo in strength conditioning during the eighties and the nineties. Fortunately, this is starting to change; especially during the last few years where more natural and functional forms of exercise are starting to become popular. Seriously, how can somebody be considered strong if he cannot even move his own body. Instead of *"bro can you even lift?"* the real question should be *"Bro, can you even lift yourself?"*

Just pick a guy out of any gym who can easily pull his own body weight in the lat pull-down machine and ask him to do the same repetitions on a pull up bar. Or pick a guy who can bench press double his bodyweight and ask him to do a one-arm push up...99.9% of them will fail. I don't know about you, but for me doing a one-arm push up on the spot is a lot cooler than claiming that you can bench press an X amount weight. Stick around long enough and we'll get to that one-arm push up before you know it!

Four Reasons Bodyweight Programs Fail People
1. Either Doing Too Little or Doing Too Much

Since I started this project, very often people come to me for advice on their bodyweight workouts. The following are usually the two main reasons they are not progressing: Either they are doing too little or they are doing too much. The first category usually adopts a bodybuilding philosophy in their bodyweight routine - such as dividing workouts into back training days, chest training days and leg training days. This training approach of training one muscle group once or twice per week will not benefit you when applied to bodyweight training (more on this later in Strength Basics).

The second category is usually doing too much. Not so much in terms of training volume, but rather in the variety of exercises. Doing a numerous variety exercises in one workout but not really going hard on any of the important exercises won't do you any good either. This is a common problem with most of the bodyweight ebooks I have read. Most of them offer people a huge overwhelming variety of bodyweight exercises. As a result, people end up doing a little bit of this, a little bit of that without focusing on the simplest, but also most important principle of strength training, Progressive Overload. Progressive Overload simply means to focus your training efforts in such a way that you continue to increase the intensity of your exercises through time (more on this in Strength Basics).

Bodyweight training, in comparison with weight lifting, may have limitations when it comes to finding a variety of high intensity functional exercises. Because there is a lot of extra fluff in terms of how many bodyweight exercises there are out there, you will have to - as Bruce Lee would simply say – "absorb what is useful and discard what is not." You need to take maximum advantage of the big muscle building bodyweight exercises. If you remember only one thing from this chapter, remember the following:

If an exercise is important, do it three times per week; if it's not, don't do it all...

2. Not Doing The Right Exercises.

If you want to get strong and build muscle you have to train using your primal movement patterns. Pull, push and squat. If you are not focusing on Pull ups, Push ups, Dips and lunges as a beginner in every bodyweight workout, you are training in vain. These multi-joint exercises give you the best bang for your buck and focusing on anything else will simply waste your time. The whole secret to bodyweight strength is to repeatedly do these exercises in every workout while keeping your rep range between 5-15 reps as you will see in point 3.

Pull, Push & Squat - The Big Muscle Building Movements

3. Tooooo Many Reps.

If you want to build muscle, science has proven that an intensity level between 70% and 90% is the most optimum range. This means that you have to use a rep range of between 5-15 reps. Applying this rep range to all the big muscle builders will recruit muscle fiber in depth and trigger anabolic hormones in the most effective way in order to build muscle and burn fat. Higher rep ranges of 20 reps can offer some extra benefits but only after you have been training seriously for at least a year. We will discus this topic more later on.

Unfortunately, most people who train with bodyweight turn their strength workouts into cardio workouts by doing push-up sets of 30 repetitions or more. If you have reached a point in an exercise where you can do 15 clean push-ups, its time to move onto a more difficult progression. If you are wondering how to increase the intensity of an exercise, I have included in the last chapter of this book enough progressions for all of the bodyweight exercises. Stick around long enough and you will be doing one arm push ups and all kinds of cool progressions in the near future.

Keep your form clean and stick between 5 and 15 repetitions

4. Not Keeping Notes.

Always write down your reps and the progression you are using. Especially in bodyweight training, it's very difficult to keep track of your progress if you don't do this. If you neglect this detail you will never get passed your newbie gains. Here is how I do it. I always note the exercise, my reps and the point after which my form started breaking down a bit.

For example: Pull ups with elastic band: 3 X [8 + 8 + (6+2)]

This means I did 3 sets of 8 repetitions. The first two sets were done with perfect form and in the third set, after the sixth rep, my form started to break down a little bit.

Quick Summary
If you want to build muscle and burn fat you have to:

1. Set aside all the extra fluff and focus on the big muscle building exercises
2. Do the important exercises three times per week
3. Focus on rep ranges between 5-15 reps
4. Keep notes

The big muscle building exercises for a beginner are:

1. Pull ups
2. Push ups
3. Weighted Lunges
4. Dips

What if you have bad genetics?

You might have noticed by now that I'm a fan of Bruce Lee. What I love most about Bruce is that he was quite ahead of his time. Even though he was a master in everything he did, Lee would always focus on perfecting the basics and simplifying what was too complex. That is the problem with most people - they forget to focus on the basics. My core value is to struggle for close to perfect results in the basics and screw the rest. Another huge influence on me is Dan John. Although I have never met him, I still consider him to be one of my mentors. His book, *"Never Let Go"* changed my life. I should probably read it again now that I'm thinking about it... Even nowadays, when my progress hits a plateau, I know I have been neglecting the basics. This is one of the most simplistic, but also the greatest insights, I have gained training these last couple of years.

I might have developed a better than average physique, yet I don't consider my results something out of anybody's reach. People around me tend to say things to me such as, "I just have good "genetics," or "I don't need to train hard to stay or get in good shape and that's why my home-workout is so effective." Yes, there are people who have to work harder than the average population to achieve the same results. And yes, there also are people with good genetics who work less for achieving the same goals. Personally, I belong to the average population when it comes to exercise genes. Most of us unfortunately are not the unique snowflake we think we are, either that's being gifted with a perfect six-pack from the fitness-fairy or cursed by the evil diet-witch with broken metabolisms.

The sum total of the life you have been living till now is what has made you what you are. Accept it and instead of complaining that you want to make a change, take action.

As an athlete, I was always the typical guy in the team who trained the hardest, following my coach's advice to the letter. Still, I had average results and ended up not having a chance when competing with the pair of guys on my team who were blessed with great genetics. I never had that, and just like most of us, I have always worked hard for my results.

As to body composition, that's another excuse I have been hearing all my life. Things like "you eat all you want and still stay ripped" and "it's in your genes to stay skinny" are excuses I have heard from people around me all my life. Talking is a lot easier than doing. Because I heard this one so often, I started believing that I am probably blessed with good body composition. I thought that I could probably eat a bit more than others without gaining as much fat. When I started this project and delved deeper into the field of nutrition and exercise, I decided to test this theory. The basic reason people gain weight is because they consume more calories than they burn (duuuh).

So, for three and a half months I tracked my calories to extreme detail and kept close watch on my weight. I ate the exact amount of calories my body burned according to a very accurate formula for tracking caloric needs. Besides "clean" foods", my diet also included stuff like ice-cream and chocolate up to 15% of my total caloric intake. Results? After eating the exact amount of calories my body required for three and a half months, I gained... two hundred grams! Two hundred grams is an insignificant amount of weight and means that my weight remained stable. This simply confirms that I belong to the typical average male of my age and I do not have magic metabolism. Trust me, I wish I did...I'd be probably eating a bucket of ice-cream while writing this paragraph.

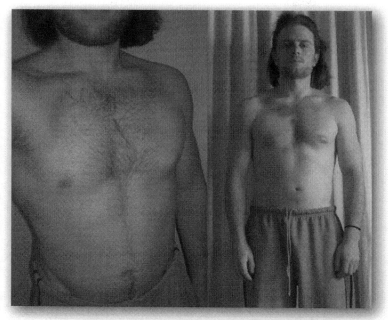

(Four years after my accident and an unhealthy lifestyle)

The years that followed my accident took a great a toll to my body. Being in and out of hospitals for five years, being operated on a total of thirteen times, consuming huge amounts of antibiotics all those years and being in a stressed and depressed mental state for so long was detrimental. From being in fantastic shape as a competitive athlete, I ended up becoming what people call "skinny fat" (lack of muscle tissue in combination with excessive fat). My whole body looked weak and sick and my stomach was constantly bloated. The good thing out of this experience was that I was able to start building my physique from scratch and I can give you an unbiased picture of my progress and results.

Along the way I made a lot of mistakes, but I also learn a great deal from them. I have made several adjustments in the training programs I have today in my book and I believe that you can make even more progress using these programs in their current, perfected state.

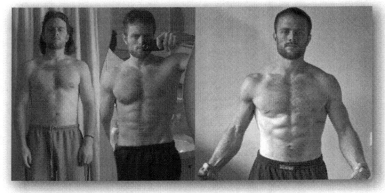

My progress after 1.5 year of training with HomeMade Muscle

3

Why train at home?

WHEN I FIRST started training at home, it was mostly out of necessity and for personal reasons. Nowadays, having a couple of thousand subscribers on my YouTube channel and people in general reaching out to me who find my work helpful and motivating, is something that has become a very powerful inspiration for me to keep on working on my HomeMade Muscle project. Training at home every day gives me more and more insight to improve this project while implementing it with all kinds of other topics that I study. Even if it wasn't for all the above, I still would not consider switching to a gym workout program. Once you know how to effectively train in the comfort of your own house, it can become incredibly convenient and suitable to your lifestyle. I don't know about you, but I love convenience.

Here are some typical advantages of training at home:

- Not having to plan going to the gym, taking a bus or the car, looking for a parking spot, etc.
- Not packing a big gym bag and worrying about forgetting something (growing up as an athlete, I always hated this)
- Not undressing and changing clothes with weird dudes in the locker room
- No smelling people in your face
- Not sitting in someone else's sweat or worrying about athletes foot in the showers
- No waiting in line for busy exercise equipment, such as the bench press
- No one to hassle you about lifetime memberships or rules
- No Christina Aguilera playing loudly while you're trying to concentrate and get in those last two reps.

My Favorite Reasons For Training at Home
1.HomeMade Muscle will save you a lot of Money

The first and most obvious advantage of training at home is not paying for a gym membership and expensive equipment. Home bodyweight workouts have only two requirements: 1) gravity; and 2) your own body. The only equipment I strongly advise you to get in the beginning is a pull up bar. Pull ups are the king of strength exercise when it comes to the upper body. If you think of all the money you will be saving yourself from gym membership fees just by spending $20 bucks for a pull up bar - trust me you are making a wise investment.

2. HomeMade Muscle workouts will save you a lot of Time

The most common excuse I hear from people who don't exercise is that they don't have time. Well, training in your own house, besides saving you money, also saves you a lot of time. Think about it, if you calculate all the time you need to pack a gym bag, travel all the way to the gym, change in the locker room, wait for your turn on crowded exercise machines and then all of that in reverse, it usually costs most people at least an extra hour or two. Training in the comfort of your own house means no commuting, no need for looking for a parking space and no need to unpack big gym bags of sweaty clothes. Once you are finished training in your home, you can immediately take a nice hot shower in your own bathroom, wear dry clothes and kick-back, or do whatever else you have to do. This program requires, on average, 3 training hours per week which is time well worth spending by anyone for the reward of a healthier, stronger and leaner body.

3. HomeMade Muscle is Psychotherapy

One of the things I love most when training at home is that you can really let go. You can express all of the frustration and aggression that bottles up during the rest of the day at work, school or wherever. You can scream through those last reps, curse, yell and generally express whatever emotions you are going through that day or that phase of your life! (Try though not to do this late at night, you don't want your neighbor calling the police thinking you are strangling someone). This has a great calming affect once you finish training. It may sound weird to some and others will totally understand what I'm talking about. I consider it as a kind of catharsis. A lot of times, training for me is more psychotherapy than exercise. Just give it a try and you will understand. People nowadays keep too much emotion bottled up in them and expressing these emotions through physical exertion gives the body and mind a great relief.

Ah, home sweet home, where your own personal gym is always open, twenty-four hours a day and three hundred and sixty five days a year. The speakers are playing Rihanna... wait what? I mean the speakers are playing Survival by Eminem or Burning Heart by Survivor, the air smells the way you like it to smell and the water in the shower is always warm.

Advantages of Bodyweight Training
From Michael Boyle's fantastic book - Advances in Functional Training

> "Technique, Technique,. Technique. Never compromise. Use bodyweight when possible and practical. Do lots of push-ups, fee-elevated push-ups, one-leg squats, chin-ups and dips. Bodyweight exercises are humbling. Not only will athletes learn to respect their bodyweight, but they will also see the value of these easy exercises."

From Easy Strength by Dan John and Pavel Tsatsouline

> "Pull-ups not only build the pulling muscles but also develop the abs. I dare you to find someone who can do 20 strict reps and does not have rockhard abs. Use many pull-up variations: change grips, do pull-ups off ropes and rings, etc"

I expect people to be excited when I motivate and tell them that they can get in great shape in the comfort of their own home spending only $20 bucks on a pull up bar. Unfortunately, most of them just look at me in disbelief. It probably sounds too good to be true or they have tried getting in shape with some other promising easy home workout plan that didn't work.

Gym Machines vs. Bodyweight

Unfortunately, most of us have been mislead into believing that in order to get in shape we need all those shiny complicated machines we see in big corporate gyms with touch screens and all sort of other gizmos on them. Some of them feel as if you are using some fighting machine to battle against aliens. The truth is that battling ehm.. I mean exercising only with machines and focusing too much on isolation movements can lead to developing a dysfunctional body. There is lack of development in stabilizing muscles in our body's connective tissue. As a result, there is no functional strength and people are more prone to injury.

On the other hand, mastering your own bodyweight requires:

- Multi-joint exercises that activate multiple muscle groups
- Analogous development of muscles with their connective tissues
- Superior core activation in comparison with gym type machines

- Balance improvement
- Coordination improvement
- Kinesthetic awareness

Kinesthetic awareness is your body's knowledge of your surroundings which you receive via the sensory receptors in your joints, muscles and skin. Also, those of you who are wondering if they are missing a lot from not doing isolation exercises, keep in mind that multi-joint exercises are more effective in producing an anabolic hormonal stimulus for muscle hypertrophy than small scale / single joint isolation type exercises.

Practicality: Bodyweight exercises can be done almost anywhere with minimum equipment.

Awesomeness Factor: Bodyweight exercises are a much more entertaining and motivational way to develop strength. Instead of striving to add that extra plate of weight every month, your goal is to perform cooler and more impressive movement variations. Once advanced bodyweight exercises can be performed with good form and ease, they can provide great visual appeal. Think about it, what is more awesome and fun...talking about how much weight you can bench press at the gym or performing a one arm push up at the beach while making it seem easy?

After all the training systems I have tried in my life, I always conclude that bodyweight exercise makes me stronger and keeps my body and mind healthier...

Is This Program For You?

Bodyweight training can be quite challenging especially for heavy people and people who haven't previously done any kind of strength exercise in their life. For this reason, I have included progressions for every exercise in order to help you gradually ease into them. There are multiple easier progressions to start from until you are strong enough to perform the basic form of the exercise. Plus, I also have extra advanced variations for when you grow even stronger. So, regardless of your sex, current physical condition and your weight, if you stick to the guidelines in this book you won't have any problems.

What If I'm Too Heavy?

Just to be realistic and not BS you, keep in mind that excessive fat can get in the way of this program if you want to get the most out of it. Think about it, if you weigh 300 pounds and you are trying to perform a handstand push-up it would be the equivalent of trying to push more than 330 pounds on an overhead shoulder-press machine. No matter how strong you become, it will be pretty difficult to attain such a high level of strength and you will be stuck in the simple progressions of some exercises probably forever.

My advice to overweight people is to combine HomeMade Muscle workouts with a proper diet in order to lose as much excessive fat as possible. Besides being more efficient at bodyweight exercises, losing weight and getting closer to a 12% body fat (for men) will help your physiology to maximize muscle hypertrophy and decrease fat storage. In simple words, your body will be able to build muscle and burn off fat faster.

What If I'm Too Strong For It?

Moving to the other end of the spectrum, if you believe you are too strong for bodyweight exercises don't rush too quickly to such a conclusion before you can perform all the advanced variations of the exercises with perfect form. Personally, I'm not at that point either. Just trying to perfect your form can have a major impact on increasing the difficulty of an exercise. So set your ego aside and focus on good form before you think you are too good for bodyweight exercise.

> *"He who conquers others is strong; he who conquers himself is mighty"*
>
> - Lao-tzu

4

What you need to know about
strength training

IN ORDER TO become stronger, your body needs three things: Stress, Recovery and Adaptation. This means that your muscles should be **stressed** enough in order to understand that next time the same stress occurs they must be stronger to handle it more efficiently. Once stress is applied to our neuromuscular system, an appropriate amount of time is required in order for our body to **recover**. If stress is re-applied too soon, strength development will happen at a slower rate. Therefore, thanks to the ability of the human body to **adapt** and become stronger in order to survive, we can manipulate stress (in our case, stress provided by bodyweight exercises) in order to become stronger and develop a more aesthetic physique. In fact, the main reason our species has survived till this point in time, is mainly thanks to how gifted we are in this whole process of adaptation.

Of course, there are limitations and different rates in which adaptation occurs. For example, if you're a complete novice in strength training you will build muscle and strength a lot faster than someone who has been training for two years. So even though a beginner might add one or two pull ups every week, this doesn't mean that this will continue to happen at the same rate. Think about it, if you begin doing 3 pull ups and add just one pull up every week, within a year, which is about 52 weeks, you will be able to do 55 pull ups. In two years you will be able to do more than 200 pull ups. Sorry to disappoint, but that's not how it works (if only).

As obvious as this is, a lot of people, and especially beginners, tend to ignore this point. So did I when I started lifting weights at the age of 15. Man, I thought, if I continue adding 10 kilos to my bench press every month I'll be a beast before I'm even 18!

As a forewarning, the rest of this chapter may be somewhat technical and clinical in nature. So, those of you who don't have a background in exercise science or haven't read any other strength related books might get a tiny bit bored by learning words like eccentric and isometric contraction. Still, I need you to have a basic understanding of these concepts so that we can communicate more efficiently throughout the remainder of the book and so that you can get the best value and results out of it.

What is Strength?

Strength is the foundation from which all forms of athletic movement becomes possible. A solid strength foundation should be the first and most important element in someone's exercise program. If your goal is simply to develop an aesthetic physique, strength training in combination with a proper diet is all you need. Not that cardio is bad or cannot aid your goals if done strategically, but it's not necessary (more on this later).

Our muscles are governed by our nervous system, which is operated by our brain. Together, our muscles and our nervous system form our neuromuscular system. These two are always interconnected; think of them like electricity and magnetism - you cannot have the one without the other. Therefore, whenever you apply stress on your muscles, whether you are doing pull-ups or weighted lunges, you also apply stress on your nervous system. Both of them can only handle so much. If you over-train them for a long period, they will eventually start to fatigue and the overall amount of reps you can perform on a daily basis will decline.

Types of Muscle Tension
Strength is produced by our muscles with three types of tension:

1. Concentric Tension: This is when the muscle "belly" decreases in size to produce force. To remember this type, think that the muscle always contracts in the concentric type. Keep in mind that in all three situations the muscles contract but most people have in mind concentric tension when they think about muscle contraction.

2. Eccentric Tension: Is when the muscle belly increases in size while the muscle is contracting. To remember this, think that the muscle extends when the muscle is in eccentric contraction.

3. Isometric Tension: Is when the length of the muscle remains the same while still producing tension. Iso in Greek means equal.

If it's the first time you are hearing of these terms you might feel overwhelmed. Hey, when I first heard them I was more than overwhelmed. But, have a look at the following examples which will clear up any confusion:

Concentric Contraction Examples
Concentric contraction is when the muscle produces tension while it's decreasing in size.

- When you are pulling yourself up by doing a chin up, your biceps are contracting concentrically;
- When you are pushing yourself up during a push up, your chest is again contracting concentrically; and
- When you are pushing yourself up during a weighted lunge, your quadriceps are once again performing a concentric contraction.

Eccentric Contraction Examples
Eccentric tension occurs when, as we said previously, the muscle decreases in size. In eccentric contraction our muscles are used as brakes so that we have better control over the movement.

- When you are lowering your body down from the top point of a chin up, your biceps act like brakes to control the movement and make it smoother;
- When you are lowering yourself down during a push up, your triceps are performing a concentric contraction.

Isometric Examples:

Isometric tension happens when the muscle produces tension while the joints around it remain in a fixed position. Whenever you are flexing your guns (biceps) in pride, while keeping your elbows steady, you are performing an isometric contraction. Isometric contraction is used mainly for stability and balance purposes. Here are some more examples of isometric contractions:

- If you pull yourself up in a chin up and remain at the top position, your biceps are contracting isometrically;
- If you remain on the top or bottom position of a push-up, your triceps are again contracting isometrically; and
- If you stand on the tip of your toes on one leg, your calf muscle is contracting isometrically.

Don't worry if you are still struggling to fully understand the differences between these contractions, its completely normal. Add a bookmark on this page and refer to it whenever you stumble upon these terms in the remainder of the text. As you read more examples in this book, you will gain a better understanding of them.

Positive and Negative Phases of a Repetition

Each repetition has a positive and negative phase. The positive phase of the repetition is when the muscle is contracting eccentrically (reducing its belly length). In a chin up for example, the positive phase is when you are pulling yourself up. During this motion, the bicep muscles contract, becoming shorter. The negative phase of the repetition is when the muscle elongates (lengthens). In the chin up, the negative phase is when you lower yourself down and straighten your arms.

An easy way to remember this is to keep in mind that the negative phase of a repetition is easier than the positive phase. So if you are doing a push, for example, and you want to figure out which is the negative phase, ask yourself: Which is the easiest part of the movement? The correct answer is the lowering phase.

Important Tip: Although the positive phase produces most of the muscle growth in an exercise, keep in mind that the negative phase (eccentric contraction) is also responsible for a significant part of it. Focusing on the negative rather than the positive phase is also another important factor in bodyweight exercise. You don't have to overdo it as some people believe; however you need to be actively controlling the movement while you are lowering your weight instead of letting gravity doing the work for you.

How Many Reps Should I Do?

If you want to become strong and lean you need to build as much muscle mass as possible. Some people tell me oh well I don't want to look like a bodybuilder. Don't worry, getting that swollen without steroids look is almost impossible. Even if you do reach a size that you are happy with that you want to maintain, just watch your diet and calorie intake and you'll be fine. It takes a lot of food to continue to grow after a certain point. After 2-3 years of serious work, once you have reached your genetic potential, muscle gains become slower and slower.

The more muscle mass you have the easier it becomes to stay lean. Keep in mind that there are also important nutritional parameters for this to happen which are discussed in the nutritional part of the book. When it comes to getting big, this is the most important thing you need to know.

Stronger is Bigger

Say that once again and don't forget it - Stronger is Bigger. This is the most important lesson I have learned from strength training while trying to gain muscle size. When you increase the strength of a muscle, whether you are using lower rep range (1-6 reps) or a higher rep range (7-20 reps), the muscle will always get bigger. There is however a prerequisite for this - you also need enough calories to facilitate the additional muscle growth. This is especially true if you're a skinny guy, if you are trying to get stronger and bigger but you are not eating a bit more from what your body needs just to preserve its weight (calorie maintenance), your body won't have enough energy to build additional muscle. It's not as if you will be building additional tissue out of thin air.

You might think that your body will use all your fat down to the last drop in order to build the extra muscle. That is not true. Yes, you can slowly build muscle and continue to lose fat if you are doing everything down to the letter, however the more you go lower than 10% body fat the more difficult and slower this process takes. Your body sees going lower than that as a threat to your existence. This is how your body thinks when you are losing too much fat: "What if I don't have enough fat to survive the following winter or the next time there will be food scarcity? I better save some of this fat and go easy on the muscle building..."

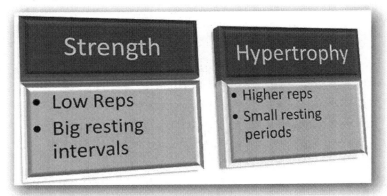

Traditional (outdated) approach to Strength & Hypertrophy

Still, there are many approaches out there towards **hypertrophy** (muscle cell growth).The most typical approach is the bodybuilder's approach, where training focuses on higher reps (12-20) with brief resting periods (usually 20-50 seconds). By now you are probably asking, "So which is it dude? Should I do low reps or high reps to get big?" If you want to get big in the most effective way possible, the answer is BOTH. The latest scientific research shows that you need a good strength foundation based on low reps to build on a higher rep range in order to build muscle mass in the most effective way. Homemade Muscle serves that goal by always starting you with five reps and focusing on building that up to 15. Once you reach 15 reps you move to a higher progression starting from 5 reps again.

Why Low Reps Are Important

Our neuromuscular system, as described previously is the functional integrated whole of our body's nerves and muscles. Training with low reps helps improve this relationship by increasing the way our muscles communicate with our nervous system. This helps stimulate our muscles in more depth during exercise. Using our neuromuscular system with such efficacy builds an ideal foundation for muscle growth.

To use a more scientific terminology: Low rep ranges improve muscle recruitment, which is defined as the number of motor units (motor neurons integrated to muscle fibers) activated in the muscle and generating force during contraction. Due to this and the increase of contractile proteins created in muscle cells, low rep ranges play a big role in muscle hypertrophy. Especially when it comes to beginners.

To make a long and sciency sentence short: You need to become stronger if you want to be bigger...

Why Bodybuilding Reps Are Also Important

A traditional bodybuilding rep range is also essential for getting big. After all, it's how the majority of people did it in the past. High rep ranges (8-15 reps) cause our muscles to store additional glycogen. Glycogen is, in simple words, liquid muscle sugar. It is the main fuel used by the muscles in high rep ranges and it contributes to the increase in our muscle's size. However because high rep range training lacks a strength foundation, it might explain why some athletes such as lightweight power-lifters can lift heavier weights than bodybuilders.

If you want to get big, you need to take advantage of a broad rep range.

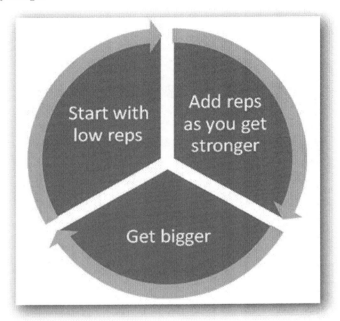

How Often Should I Train?

The main consensus on training frequency in the weightlifting world, according to science, ranges between training a muscle group 2-3 times per week, leaning mostly towards 2 times.

Now even though this might be accurate in the weightlifting world, it's not something you can copy & paste in a bodyweight program. A weightlifting program in comparison to a bodyweight program has only one advantage; you can go heavier on leg training using bilateral barbell squats, which, at the same time will tax the whole body. You see, a heavy barbell squat does not only train the lower body but it also puts a large amount of load on your upper body that has to stabilize the weight. Weighted lunges are great but they fail to place the same amount of intensity on the legs. Due to this, using a whole body workout with a frequency of three times per week in bodyweight training is a lot more efficient. You can also train effectively using a higher training frequency. But in order to avoid burning out your neuromuscular system, this type of training requires a basic amount of experience and knowledge, as well as discipline. To create such program and apply it successfully requires periodization.

Periodization in simple words is a training program that has been planned in advance for a long period of training. The aim is to reach the best possible performance using progressive cycling of bigger resting periods like deloading weeks, different training volumes and training intensities. This is used in the advanced program included in this book.

How Many Sets Should I do?

For a complete beginner, 2-3 sets seems to provide the greatest results. Still, this is not absolute because it depends on how much the individual pushes himself. In addition, muscle groups like legs for example seem to tolerate an increased training volume. As we mentioned previously when someone passes the beginners phase, his adaptive capacity becomes more advanced to the point where progress does not happen from workout session to workout session but is accumulative. The gym and the bodyweight world differ significantly in this area since bodyweight exercises such as handstand push-ups or one-arm push-ups require great technique - neuromuscular efficiency. Factors such as coordination, balance and kinesthetic awareness are part of performing these exercises properly and therefore increased training volume and frequency strategically play a great role in breaking training plateaus in bodyweight exercise.

> ***Kinesthetic awareness is*** *your body's awareness of your surroundings, which you receive via the sensory receptors in your joints, muscles & skin.*

Since most of us are not gymnasts who have been working on these abilities since we were six years old, we need a lot of practice to improve them. Increasing training frequency and training volume by reducing a bit of intensity can help the advanced bodyweight trainee to continue to improve. Increasing these abilities will also increase strength which will eventually lead to more muscle mass. Remember - Stronger is bigger. However, as previously said, this should be done strategically with an organized training program. Providing adequate rest for the neuromuscular system and joints from time-to-time by using strategies, such as de-loading weeks, is essential.

How Long Should I Rest?

The classic guidelines for muscle hypertrophy in the bodybuilding world recommend short resting periods. Although, literature doesn't have any basis to support this theory just yet, based upon both personal experience, and rest, in the anecdotal consensus out there, I believe there is some benefit in small resting periods for means of hypertrophy. Internationally renowned hypertrophy expert and scientist - Brad Schoenfeld (who has also won natural bodybuilding titles) says there isn't enough evidence yet to draw concrete conclusions on this topic but shorter resting periods increase metabolic stress, which is known to stimulate muscle remodeling. For these reasons, I have concluded that shorter resting periods used once a week in the advanced program can add some value in the training program. Plus, it also helps to make your workouts a bit more fun.

In the rest on the book I consider it important to take your time when you rest between sets until your body feels ready. I do recommend specific resting periods for practical reasons (like saving time) yet it's important to also trust your own body. From general experience and due to the fact that beginners don't have enough experience to stress their body close to its highest potential, I recommend relatively short breaks of one minute in the beginners phase. Later on in the advanced phase, once the trainee has more experience, it's important to get adequate rest in order to perform every set feeling recharged and using good form (2-3 three minutes is usually enough for this purpose). Still, these resting periods aren't meant for you to login to your Facebook with your mobile device to catch up on your notification - Stay focused!

Training Plateaus

If you complete a whole year of bodyweight strength training, remaining faithful to your program, progress will be slower and slower, just as in any strength program. As said previously you can't continue adding a pull up each week up to infinity. That's not how the body works.

There will be periods in which you will experience great improvement in your workouts and your body's physique. These periods are usually followed by plateaus. Unless you are a beginner, your progress in strength exercise will never be gradual. You advance with sudden jerks and starts. Then you may remain stationary for a while. In some cases, especially after your second year, you might even regress a tiny bit! You may strive hard for a long period of time and not see any progress. Then one day when you least expect it, you suddenly start ascending again. Many people get discouraged on these long periods of stagnation and think that the workout plan they are using is not good or is not effective anymore. So they take the easy way out - they quit!

It is crucial to learn to recognize these plateaus and have the emotional intelligence required to stay faithful to your program. Plateaus are natural... This means that you are no longer a beginner and that you have taken your workouts seriously. Long periods of no progress can be tiring mentally and physically, so you must remain patient and develop mental toughness during these times. What you can achieve is strictly up to you. When it comes to health and fitness goals, it does not matter if you have the best personal trainer and the best nutritionist in the world. If you are missing a strong will, all else will crumble. As my bro Bruce would say:

> *"If you always put limits on everything you do,*
> *physical or anything else, it will spread into your*
> *work and into your life. There are no limits. There*
> *are only plateaus, and you must not stay there,*
> *you must go beyond them."*

- Bruce Lee

Overtraining

Recovery depends on multiple factors including how much time you rest between your workouts. Recently, a guy named CT Fletcher became popular on YouTube. CT, who is probably the most motivational exercise figure I have ever seen, promotes the "There **is** no overtraining" approach to exercise in many of his videos. A lot of people take it literally, criticize him, blame him for lying on steroid use, etc., etc... What do I think? Well I won't get into the whole steroid thing, but I will focus on what matters; overtraining definitely exists. If you overdo it, you will harm your progress and your body. Still, I think CT gets a very important message across. His message is that there are too many lazy people and keyboard warriors out there, afraid to push themselves a bit and talking shit while eating bon bons (as CT puts it) instead of getting their lazy ass of the couch (as he says). Some people just need figures like CT to wake up. I don't believe he is being literal by saying there is no overtraining and I'm sure if you read his workout books there will be some kind periodization in his training programs. So don't take people like him literally, avoid extremes and if it helps you - use these people to get pumped up and motivated.

Recovery

Aside from the exercise/resting ratio, there are also some other very important factors that influence recovery and strength performance. Remember, our muscles grow while we are resting. Three important factors to take under consideration for a proper recovery in strength development are the following:

<u>1. Sleep Quality and Quantity</u>

Sleep quality and quantity. Our DNA hasn't changed much in the last 10.000 years and that means that our biological clock works optimally in the same natural rhythms as our ancient ancestors. Our bodies are programmed to sleep according to the circadian cycle which basically means that we are programmed to sleep when there is darkness and wake up when there is light. Studies have shown that there might even be a connection of bad sleep with diabetes, obesity and depression.

Sleep is probably the most important factor for strength athletes in terms of recovery. Getting an average of 8 hours of quality sleep (30-60 more minutes if you are in your teens) is a natural way to supplement your exercise program with anabolic hormones. Proper hormonal secretion depends highly on having a proper sleep cycle. Hormones like Testosterone and the Growth Hormone are highly associated with proper sleep and play a big role in muscle recovery.

Sleeping Tips:

My approach for getting quality sleep is to always get in bed early and stay there for at least eight hours. There are periods when I don't actually sleep many of those hours, however I still make it a habit to always rest during that time span.

In the winter when there is less light I go to bed around 10:00 p.m., read for about half an hour and sleep (or lay there) until at least 6:30 a.m. If you have trouble sleeping early, reading in bed is the best solution I have found to solve this problem. The second best is 15-20 minutes of mindfulness meditation prior to nap time.

Never eat a big heavy meal prior to going to bed unless you like nightmares and restless sleep. If you eat dinner late at night, either make sure you eat a moderate-small portion of food, or if you eat a big meal like me, do it at least three hours before.

2. Physical & Mental Relaxation When You Are Not Training or Sleeping.

When you are too stressed mentally for long periods of time, your body's capability to build muscle optimally might be hindered. Your body will be over-producing stress related hormones, such as cortisol, which reduce the production of opposite anabolic hormones (like Testosterone and Growth Hormone) which help your body recuperate and build bigger and stronger muscles. You may think, "Ok bro, this is all good but I cannot command my mind not to be stressed or depressed, can I?" Yes you can and this brings me to my next tip:

Meditation

Exercise, in combination with meditation and a daily dose of sunlight on top of that, is the best way to naturally fight stress and depressive moods. Personally, besides exercising, I also meditate every day which has made a huge difference in my stress levels and has also improved the quality of my thoughts, making me a more positive person. Meditation has clinically shown to have the following effects:

- Reduces blood pressure
- Stress reduction

- Improves sleep quality
- Strengthens the immune system
- Makes us react more calm in stressful situations
- Might help us against premature aging
- Improves concentration

The type of meditation that works for me is mindfulness meditation but there are many types of meditation out there, each suitable for everyone's idiosyncrasies. Here are some different forms of meditation:

- Mindfulness
- Bioenergetics and dancing meditation
- Sound meditation
- Body awareness meditation
- Chanting meditation

And the list goes on...

If you are interested, just find a good book on the type of meditation that seems most appealing to you and begin practicing every day. As shown in studies even as little as 15 minutes per day can make a difference!

Personal Trick to Stop Stressing Over Useless Stuff: Whenever I find myself stressing over trivial matters, I have a personal trick to relax myself. I visit the future elderly version of me. I imagine him laid on a bed, wrinkled and having just a few more days to live. The moment I see myself through his eyes, stressing over the insignificant matters that are burdening me, I realize how unimportant it all is and that life is too short to pay attention to such things. Try it; you'll be surprised at how much it can help at times.

3. Sunlight

Many people suffer from symptoms of seasonal affective disorder during the winter months. This is believed to be closely correlated with lack of sunlight exposure. Sunlight exposure can benefit mood by boosting levels of key hormones and also by producing vitamin D. Vitamin D is produced in the liver and kidneys from precursor chemicals that are synthesized in the skin, when UV rays from the sun shine on it.

Despite the limited evidence available currently, athletes and trainers in the early 20th century believed that UVB radiation was beneficial to athletic performance. Accumulating evidence supports the existence of a functional role for vitamin D in skeletal muscle with potentially significant impacts on both the performance and injury profiles of young, otherwise healthy athletes. While further research is required to evaluate the level of vitamin D required for optimal muscular function, my personal experience says that getting 15 minutes of sunlight on a daily basis (ideally somewhere after your workout) can help you recover more efficiently. Consider this my bro tip.

Excuses

For the last couple of months while I have been training, the noise from a bar on the lower level of my house has been interfering with my sleep quality. Two to three times per week my sleeping quality sucks and there are days when I see it affecting my workouts. I feel heavier. Still, I pay my dues and follow my workout plan. My point here is that if you wait for the perfect conditions in life they will never come. You will always have at least some stress in your life, you might live in a country with not enough sunlight or you might have a kid that keeps waking you up late at night. Try to get the best out of your current situation and find a way to get your workout done. The only bad workout is the one that doesn't happen.

5

Abs
The holy grail of fitness

I'M NOT A BIG fan of the expression - abs are made in the kitchen. Sure, its 50% true, but in order to lose fat and reveal the abdominal area you also need to train it. Abs are just like any other skeletal muscle. They are a striated, skeletal muscle group, which means that you need to work on them 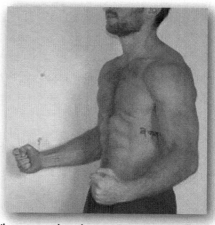 at least two times a week. Where people take a wrong approach to ab training is using the wrong exercises and overdoing it. On the right you can see is a picture of me last summer (2014).

If you zoom in on it you can see that the upper part of my abs extends even more than my chest, so you could say my abs were quite defined during that time period. Also, I had a very low body fat percentage which, besides helping me look really ripped, also cost me some muscle loss; with my chest looking flatter than ever. During that period, the only direct ab-work I did was Dragon Flags. However, notice that I say direct work since I was doing a hell of a lot of bodyweight exercise.

How Much Abs is Healthy?

The first and most important thing I want to mention on this topic is that having a six-pack isn't per se equivalent to being healthy. Once you start going lower than 11-12% body fat (21-22% for women) and start moving closer to 6% body fat (13% for women) you are likely doing more harm than good to your health. Of course keep in mind that people are different due to genetic factors and while some can feel great at 8% others might feel weak and even sick.

I'm not saying you shouldn't try getting ripped if that is your goal. But, if your face is starting to look way too edgy, or if, besides your abdominal area, the rest of your physique starts to look worse and if other related problems start occurring; like experiencing a low libido, if you're a guy, or having menstrual issues, if you're a woman, these are good signs that you are probably doing more harm than good.

Abs tend to be a topic people obsess on a lot. Since the abdominals are part of a bigger unit - the core, I will also mention some important points about the core in general. First, let's start with two of the most common myths when it comes to abdominal training...

The Truth About Ab Training

Although these myths are finally starting to fade from the fitness industry, I feel it's important to make sure that everybody who reads this article knows the following two myths about abdominal and core training:

1. Doing hundreds of abdominal exercise repetitions every day won't help you build a strong ripped stomach! Your abs are anatomically just as any other muscle which means that you don't need to train them more than three times a week. You need to use high intensity and a rep range of 1-15 repetitions per set. Overtraining your abs, as many people do especially by doing a lot of crunches, can only cause you problems like back pain as we will see later on.

2. Abdominal exercises burn fat around your stomach! There is no direct metabolic pathway from your abdominal musculature to the fat tissue surrounding it. In order to burn fat and convert it to energy, your body must first send the fat to your liver where it will be broken down to fatty acids. This fat comes from all over your body. Gender, age and genetics are responsible for determining which areas are going to be more "preferred" as fat sources. For example, if you are the "chicken-leg" body type, while you are doing ab crunches your body might be burning more fat from your legs!

A guy named Ged Musto, performed 1,555 Unaided Sit-Ups in 30 minutes in 2005 which was an Official British and World Record.

If you Google him or check out his YouTube vids, his abs just look like they simply belong to a guy that simply works out - nothing really special though.

Remember that abs are just like all the other muscles you train. You need muscle tension. If you are doing more than 15 - 20 reps per set, you are doing too many!

Three basic points to keep in mind when pursuing abs:

- **You have to get rid of the extra fat.** Although strength exercise can tone your abs and help you burn some extra calories, it's only gonna get you half way there. The other 50% is diet which will play the biggest role in revealing them. Your abs may be even more defined than Stallone in Rocky 3 but if you never burn the fat around them they will never be visible.
- **It won't happen at the same speed for everyone.** Genetics play a big role. Some people just have a harder time getting a ribbed stomach because they tend to store more fat around the stomach due to their body type. If you belong in this group of people then unfortunately you need to have greater patience.
- **Leaner doesn't always mean healthier.** If you pass the point of 8-10% body fat and continue to drop weight, keep in mind that you will also start losing a significant amount of muscle tissue and you can create hormonal imbalances that can lead to further problems.

The Big Crunch

A lot of people base their ab work on the thought that the basic function of the abdominal muscles is movement production. If you study anatomy & kinesiology you will see that a significant role of the abdominal musculature is actually to prevent motion and to keep your lumbo-pelvic region (lower back) more stable.

Are crunches causing you back pain?

Typical floor crunches train mostly the upper part of your rectus abodminis, which most of the time is already too tight. Dr. Stuart M. McGill a Professor of Spine Biomechanics and one of the most famous scientists on this topic. After studying how the spine works for more than three decades, Dr. McGill has come to loathe sit-ups. It doesn't matter whether they are the full sit-ups beloved by military trainers or the crunch versions so ubiquitous in gyms. "What happens when you perform a sit-up is that the spine is flexed into the position at which it damages sooner."

My Favorite Ab Exercises

The following are my 2 favorite and only targeted exercises for ab training.

1. Dragon Flags. Your rectus abdominis (six-pack) in combination with your external obliques (side abs) act as stabilizing muscles which are responsible for keeping your torso aligned with your lower body. Dragon Flags are the best exercise I have encountered so far to work not only your abs, but also your whole core. Of course, this is not an easy exercise and you need to build it up very carefully. Start with leg raises and slowly through time use the progressions in the exercise menu chapter to work yourself up to the famous Dragon Flag. It personally took me a year to get 5 clean reps - so take it easy ;)

2. One arm-push ups - the side ab exercise. You might be asking, "how the hell are one arm push-ups going to work my side abs?" Besides being an awesome exercise for your shoulders, arms and chest, it's also a good rectus abdominis exercise and an even greater oblique (side ab) exercise. Your obliques need to work very hard to keep the body from rotating due to the lack of stability by balancing only on one arm. The first time I started working on one arm push ups, I woke up the next day feeling as if someone had punched me on the side of my stomach. Sure it's a difficult exercise and not ideal for beginners, but you can work on progressions and gradually build it up.

6

Stretching
Facts & Fallacies

A COMMON MYTH is that flexibility increases the length of your muscles. This is something that has been disproven a long time ago. Still most of us have experienced greater flexibility by making stretching a habit so why is this?

When we assume uncomfortable and unusual positions, like bending over to touch our toes, our muscles tend to tighten up due to protective mechanisms. Because of these mechanisms. when we try to extend our range of motion in these positions, for example when we are trying to stretch our hamstrings, we experience discomfort. What happens when we practice stretching is that our neuromuscular system becomes more accustomed to unusual positions and it learns to relax in them. This lets our muscles loosen up and as a result bigger ranges of motion are allowed in our joints.

Studies have also shown that it might cause you to get injured if done exactly before intense exercise. Some specialists still recommend it though, not directly before the main part of an exercise program but prior to warming up. Personally I like to stretch some of the tight muscles in my lower body before warming up.

To stretch or not to stretch?

Below is a list of the most common stretching myths that have been disproven by science in the last decades. Stretching research has shown that:

- Stretching is not an effective warm-up
- Stretching does not prevent delayed-onset muscle soreness (DOMS)
- Stretching does not prevent injury
- Stretching does not increase the structural length of your muscles

So, to stretch or not to stretch? That is the question...

Stretching feels good to a lot of people (including me). Also, even though research has shown that it doesn't reduce muscle soreness; a lot of people report the opposite. In my experience, sometimes it does, other times it doesn't. Very often, I just have a strong urge to stretch. It feels as if its an annoying neurological itch I just have to scratch in order to feel better. Stretches such as toe touches for hamstrings, as well as stretching muscles like the gluteus medius and piriformis in a lying position almost feels as good as a professional massage. Still, the exact science of these feelings and what might only be physiological in nature, is not yet clear in the academic world.

Here is my recommendation for stretching with HomeMade Muscle. Stretch when you feel like it and specifically, focus on the muscles that feel tight. There is no need to over-stretch your joints that are already too flexible. Doing this, for no specific reason (like being a martial artist) and without professional acquiescence might even cause hyper-mobility related problems. Avoid stretching intensely before working out. If you have the urge, just gently stretch whatever feels tight for a brief 5-10 seconds and do it a bit dynamically instead of completely statically.

I personally believe there is more to stretching than what has been discovered up until now, and in the future it will find its place in exercise science. Until then, I still like to stretch whenever it feels right. Stretching also helps me relax mentally. If you would like to dive more into the whole scientific analysis of stretching, I highly recommend you read Paul Ingraham's amazing article, "Quite a Stretch." Say hello to him from me if you pass by his website and leave a comment.

Here are some of my favorite stretches...

1. Doorway Chest & Shoulder Stretch. Stand under the middle of a doorway with one foot straddling the threshold and your hands gripping the inside of the doorway, on each side. Shift your weight on the forward foot until you feel a pull in your shoulders and chest. Keep your hands at chest height, first to focus more on the chest. After that, place your hands just above your shoulder's height, to focus more on your anterior deltoids (front part of the shoulder). To isolate arms separately, face your body a bit towards the opposite side of the arm you want to focus on.

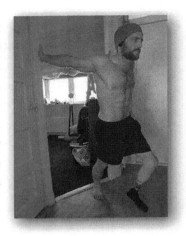

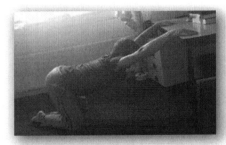

Desk Stretch for Lats and Chest. You can use your desk, a windowsill, a kitchen counter or any kind of ledge about waist high. Sit on your knees, bend over and place your hands on the surface just a bit wider than shoulder width. Gently lower your torso until you feel the stretch on your lats and chest. You can also isolate one arm at a time.

Hamstring stretch with bike tube. Using again the bike tube, an elastic band, or even a wide belt, lie on your back, keep your left leg on the floor and bend your right leg so that your foot rests flat on the floor. Loop your elastic band around the upper part of your right foot, holding onto an end of the band with each hand. Straighten your knee and pull the leg slowly towards your chest.

You will feel in a stretch in the whole back area of your right leg. Pull your leg really slow so you don't end up straining your hamstrings or anything else. Do the same for the other leg. This stretch is ideal for people with a sedentary lifestyle where these muscles tend to be quite tight.

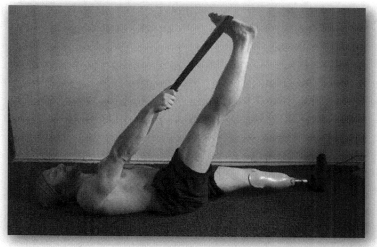

(bike tube stretch)

Piriformis & Gluteus Medius Stretch. Lie on your back, legs extended along the floor, right arm resting on the floor straight out to the side. Bring your right knee in toward your chest and very gently clasp the knee with your left hand, then gradually pull the knee over toward the floor, keeping your right arm and shoulder flat on the floor. You should feel a stretch in the hip and lower back. This can help relax muscles that cause back pain and get tight when you spend a lot of time sitting (office jobs etc).

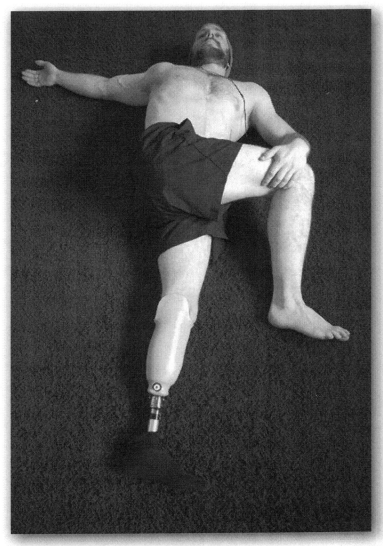

(ideal stretch for lower back tension)

7

Mobility - Use it or Lose it

A DAY CAME when my, once young and well-oiled shoulders, started feeling like the squeaky hinges of a metallic old door. Sensitive elbows, wrists and tight shoulders are common among people who abuse bodyweight training for too long. Two other factors that seem to cause these types of problems for people in general are aging and inactivity. It's easy to blame the natural process of aging for all our problems but another very important fact that contributes to joint issues is inactivity.

I did a lot of research and self experimentation with self-myofascial relief methods such as foam rolling, massage and stretching but I found out that the best way to treat this issues is the also the simplest. The best way to prevent common joint problems and also improve issues from past exercise abuse is motion. **You just need to prescribe your joints with a healthy diet of mobility drills**. Why? Simply said, **"Motion is lotion."** Joint health depends largely on repetitive healthy movement that covers all the natural ranges of motion the joint has.

Whenever somebody tells me about a new recovery or physical conditioning method, the first thing I do is to check that he is not trying to get in my wallet.

What Causes Joint Issues

Aging, imbalanced strength programs, bad exercise technique, not warming up or a combination of all of these are the usual suspects and can cause reduction of your joint's synovial fluid (which in simple words is your joint's natural lubricant). It can also cause calcium deposits and adhesions (connective tissue growth in the wrong places surrounding your joints).

Mobility vs. Flexibility

When it comes to mobility, a typical mistake is to confuse it with flexibility. Stretching for mobility is not that helpful since one does not depend on the other. You can be flexible with poor mobility and vice versa. If you want more functional joints - mobility trumps flexibility.

"Flexibility does not equal Mobility"

Joints in comparison with muscles have no direct blood supply to receive nutrients. Mobility drills improve the circulation of your joint's synovial fluid, which also helps your joints remove waste products and "smooth out" adhesions. Practicing mobility drills can restore a lot of range of motion and can help you reduce that rusty sensitive feeling your joints have as you grow older. In summary, if you want healthier and more functional joints, mobility drills are the way to go.

"Mobility trumps Flexibility"

Mobility Drills - When should I do them?

Joints such as ankles, shoulders, neck and wrists can benefit greatly from mobility drills which can help restore the joints natural range of motion. A common problem I hear from people is that they have no time to do all these "extra" healthy things. Here is how you can include mobility drills in your routine to save time. Simply replace your warm up with a full body mobility routine, add a pull and push exercise of a couple (2-3) easy sets for the upper body, a multi-joint exercise for the lower body (like squats) and you are ready to go! Other ways to include mobility drills in your schedule are as active recovery after your workout or as a separate session. Starting your day with a mobility drill can energize you in the morning or help you discharge at night before sleep. Nowadays I include my mobility drill in my exercise's warm up and some days I do them before going to bed to release some tension from my body (which also helps with sleep).

From personal experience, practicing mobility drills four times per week can make a big difference within just 21 days.

Want a video example? Go to my Youtube channel and search for "Mobility Routine - Pain-free Joint in 20 days". I've made with a basic mobility drill that covers all the basic joint movements and focuses on shoulders which are commonly-known problematic joints in people.

8

Tips for dealing with
bodyweight exercise related injury

WHEN I STARTED training again at age 27, I realized that I didn't have the same body I had in my early twenties. I'm guessing it wasn't only the age, since I wasn't that old, but also all the years of inactivity, depression and maybe even all the drugs I had to take for my leg recovery; tons of antibiotics, surgery drugs and several others.

Injury Treatment 101

When I was 20 I thought I had those indestructible "wolverine joints." Quite often I would skip doing a proper warm up and no matter what crazy stuff I would be doing, I almost never had problems. Nowadays I wish I could visit the younger version of me and tell him to slow down a little bit. Hey, I don't know about you but

I want to be that strong and a lean 65 year old tough grandpa one day. Going to the playground with my grand kids and hitting 20 chin-ups with ease while young dudes look in awe.

Keep in mind that I'm not an expert on injuries but I'll at least share with you the basics. For very mild injuries that lead to inflammation the recipe is usually simple. Elevation, Ice, Rest, Heat and Movement.

The first two days, ice the affected area every couple of hours (don't overdo it and get ice burns) and try to keep it elevated. After 48 hours, if 90% of the pain is gone, it's time for heat and some movement. When I say movement, you just want to go cautiously through the natural ranges of motion of the affected joint and later on apply some very mild stretching. All this without experiencing any pain of course. You may feel very mild discomfort but avoid anything more intense than that. Some soft massage and hot showers/baths after that are not a bad idea. Avoid working out again for at least three to four days and always go easy on your first workout.

In the following section, we will go over some of the most troublesome areas in bodyweight trainees.

Elbow, Shoulder and Wrist Pain From Straight Bar Chin-ups

A common problem strength athletes face is elbow pain. A typical reason this happens to bodyweight athletes are straight bar chin-ups. While doing chin-ups on a straight pull-up bar, your arms move in a constant fixed position, which can place unnatural stress on your joints.

Those of you who are experiencing elbow pain from chin-ups will notice that your arms and shoulders feel restriction in the lowering phase of this exercise. Especially if you lock out (straighten) your elbows. This is caused by the lack of mobility your arms have to externally rotate (that's the movement your arm does when you open a doorknob with your right hand).

To verify this do the following experiment (see image below):

1). Straighten your arm in front of you with your palm facing the floor; and 2). Slowly turn your palm towards the ceiling (rotating it externally) until it is facing it in a flat position. If you experience difficulty with keeping your palm flat while facing the ceiling, or if you cannot even flatten your palm, the chances are good that this exercise will cause you joint pain at some point if it hasn't already.

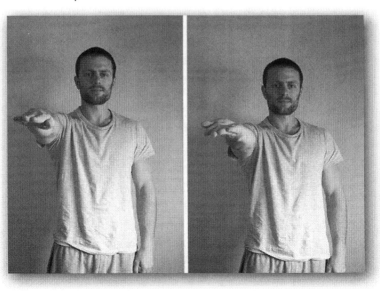

From position number 2 lift your arm vertically as if you were going to grab a bar to do chin-ups. You will observe that it becomes even more difficult to keep your palm upwards. While doing chin-ups, twisting forces are occurring inside your joints to compensate for this lack of mobility. Continuous repetition of these abusive movements will eventually cause overuse injuries.

A lack of mobility in the shoulder in combination with a lot of chin-ups over time will eventually cause some, or a combination of, the following issues:

- wrist pain
- elbow pain
- shoulder pain

Solutions & Tips

That being said, I hope I have not scared you away from chin-ups, that was that not my intention. Chin-ups are one of the best upper body exercises and they should be included in your strength exercise arsenal. Minimizing the injury potential of this exercise with the following tips will help you to keep on pounding chin-ups until you're 65 and beyond.

Tip #1 – Don't Lock Out

Always keep your elbows bent a bit while doing this exercise. Never lockout and hang on the bottom position of the reps. Don't worry, this won't hurt your gains and it will keep constant tension on your biceps, giving you a cool post-workout pump.

Tip #2 – Frequency
Don't overdo it. Six sets per week is an ideal frequency. The rest of the week use different grip varieties as mentioned below, which will also support you in doing more chin-ups and improving pulling strength in general.

Tip #3 – Grip Variety
If possible, also try to use a variety of grips. Most pull-up bars today have a neutral grip (palms facing each other) or a zig-zag grip which are friendlier for your joints. If your pull-up bar has one of these grips I would definitely prefer them over straight bar chin-ups.

Tip #4 – Don't Squeeze Too Hard!
When you squeeze your grip too hard it radiates tension up to the arm and can affect the elbow. I recommend this tip especially for people who have sensitive elbows and experience elbow pain frequently. Hold the bar more loosely and this will alleviate or prevent your elbow pain from flaring up.

Also consider some shoulder mobility exercises. These two exercises have helped me : a) **subscapularis stretch** and b) **shoulder dislocations**. If you go at my youtube channel at https://www.youtube.com/user/HomeMadeMuscles and look for "Stretch for rounded shoulders").

Ending Notes. It should go without saying, that when you are experiencing persisting pain due to chin-ups, you should first let your body heal before applying the tips above. Once you get back to your bodyweight routine, get started with a different and easier pulling exercise instead of chin-ups. Inverted rows are a good alternative. When the time is right, start gradually including chin ups back in your weekly schedule again.

Wrist Pain From Pushing Exercises

A common problem people face from bodyweight exercises is wrist pain. Too much hyperextension of the wrist in exercises like push-ups and handstands can take a toll on them.

<u>Tips for people with sensitive wrists</u>

If you have sensitive wrists, I highly recommend doing your push-ups on your knuckles. When doing knuckle push-ups, your wrists are in a neutral position and you spear them a great deal of stress (plus they look cooler). If knuckle push-ups are too difficult for you, you can always buy push up grips (or just man up and learn to do the knuckle version). Because handstand push-ups are also quite stressful for your wrists, you should also prepare your wrists before any handstand work. . Go to my youtube channel again at https://www.youtube.com/user/HomeMadeMuscles and search for Wrist & lower back warm up.

Chapter Ending Thoughts

When an injury happens, stop worrying and remember that they just are part of the game. Even when people warm up perfectly, use perfect form and eat super healthy, they still very often end up getting hurt. <u>The important thing is to find ways to minimize injury potential by figuring out what went wrong and how it could be</u>

<u>prevented</u>. A lot of people get discouraged when injuries present themselves and react very emotionally (especially if this happens in the beginning). For example, you might have just started your program and you're feeling thrilled with all the progress you've achieved after a lot of hard work. Then, suddenly when you least expect it, you get injured. You overreact and think that all the effort was for nothing. You think to yourself I might as well quit now to avoid wasting any more time or getting disappointed again in the future. The best advice I can offer is to take it easy and see these situations as a useful break for your joints and muscles to rest. You can even do some isometric exercises on the rest of the body that is not affected, if you're in the mood. Find a book on isometrics and study about it, even if it's just for fun and to keep your mind occupied.

Part 3

HomeMade Muscle Workout

1

HomeMade Muscle program structure

THE HOMEMADE MUSCLE training program consists of three training levels:

1) **Beginners**' level
2) **Basic** level
3) **Advanced** level

Even if you have trained using bodyweight exercises previously, if you haven't trained for more than two weeks I highly recommend you start from the beginner's level. This way you will avoid things like extreme soreness and injuries. Once you hit a plateau using the beginners phase, move onto the basic phase. Many beginners have the tendency to skip steps in order to "get stronger faster." This is something I also tried to do when I was a teenage rower. If only I could go 10 years back with the knowledge I now have, I could have accomplished so much more. This brings me to the classic mistake most stubborn young dudes experience when they first get started with strength training, "The Arnold fallacy".

The Arnold Fallacy

When Arnold Schwarzenegger released his training program in the seventies, everybody who wanted to develop the famous Arnold-physique bought his book. Most of them skipped the intermediate phase and used the advanced program that Arnold was using to train himself after he first invested years on mastering the basics. That didn't work well for them. Of course, I'm not comparing myself to the great Arnold, but this is a common theme in strength training.

When I was in the junior rowing team of my hometown, around the age of 15, me and a buddy of mine always tried to secretly do what the big team was doing in order to get better faster (obviously we thought we were smarter than our coach). Results? We ended up burned out.

If you are new to strength and bodyweight training, skipping the beginner's level will just result in hindering the rate of your progress. There is no need to hurry; in fact, the beginners phase is an amazing period. It's the period of the glorious "newbie gains" when building muscle and adding reps will be easier than ever. Enjoy and appreciate this time because it doesn't last long. Don't try to outsmart your body by rushing into a training phase if you haven't first done the appropriate work.

Learn to respect the basics...

The 8 Essential Bodyweight Exercises

Sculpting a lean, muscular and symmetrical physique is something I consider a form of art. What I like the most about it is that if you know how to handle the right tools it can be a form of art mastered by anyone. Of course it might seem complicated in the beginning. If you enter a huge gym for the first time you will probably become overwhelmed by the sheer volume of exercise equipment. Being completely new to strength exercise can make this experience intimidating. Something very important to learn from the beginning is that exercise quality is a lot more important than quantity.

During my journey of getting stronger, I tried almost all of the bodyweight exercises I could find out there. And trust me when I say this - there are countless of them. After doing research on a lot of bodyweight exercise books, I realized that most of them offer an endless list of exercises. Trying to mastering all of them would take a lifetime. After all, not everyone wants and can afford to train all day like a professional athlete just to look and feel good.

After a great deal of experimenting, I concluded that in order to get as strong as possible and attain an aesthetic physique I only need to use and focus on mastering 8 of them. The 8 bodyweight exercises that focus on the basic human movement patterns in the best possible way are the following:

1.   Pull-ups
2.   Push-ups
3.   Weighted lunges
4.   Dips
5.   Inverted Rows

6. Handstand Push-ups
7. Leg Raises
8. Prone Cobra

Less is more...

Keep in mind that all of these movements have progressions and advanced variations which gradually bring into play new stimulus for the body. These exercises resemble some of our most basic primal movement patterns which highly stimulate our neuromuscular system and strengthen our body's prime mover muscles in balance with your core, joints, ligaments and tendons. Trust me; if you conquer every variation of the exercises in this book you will have greater relative body strength than 99% of all people around you.

Primal Movement Patterns

Primal Movement Patterns are movements which were important for survival before man stopped living in the wild. Think about it, if you lived in the wild, would bicep curls serve great purpose in any important movements? Not really.

On the other hand, you would definitely have to climb up high surfaces which would require **pulling** yourself **up** in all kinds of different angles, according to the terrain around you.

Once you pull yourself up to chest height while climbing a surface, the next thing you have to do is to push yourself up in order to rest your chest on it. This resembles the movement used **dips** and **push-ups**.

Living in the wild would also require you to hold heavy things above your head; for example in order to build a roof for a shelter. A movement like that would require the same muscles used in **hand-stand push-ups.**

Walking across wild terrain and vegetation with your equipment/food on your back would also require movement patterns that resemble the **weighted lunge** on a daily basis. Nowadays, everybody is afraid that squats are bad for our knees. Squats are not what is causing your knees to hurt, but rather the lack of doing them. This has de-trained the proper neuromuscular pathways required to attain this position properly. Make sure you perfect the bodyweight lunge before you start adding weight.

Last, but most important of all, to perform every single one of these moves efficiently, you would need a **strong core**. No, our ancestors did not train their abs and low back muscles, because all of these muscles never atrophied and lost their integrated neuromuscular coordination in the first place. These muscles always worked in perfect sync with the rest of their body during all the movements mentioned above.

Unfortunately, our lifestyle has deeply weakened and de-trained these muscles, making us forget how to turn them on in harmony with the rest of our body when needed. Using leg raises, prone cobras and all of the exercises intergraded in this book will help you re-establish the relationship between your core and the rest of the body.

How Strong Should You Become?

The goal of the basic level is to provide you an impressive athletic physique and a realistic training program that can be performed long-term without overstressing the body's joints and ligaments. It's also ideal for people over the age of 40. It uses a three-time per week training frequency, which makes it an easy and sustainable workout plan on which you can continue to make progress steadily over time. If you're looking to become strong, healthy and look good; there is really no reason to go beyond the basic level.

Keep in mind that once you have built a significant amount of muscle with the basic level program, there is also something else you can do to do to improve your physique, even if you're just working out 1-2 times per week to maintain your progress. Improving your diet and shedding a couple of extra pounds of fat is the easiest way to look and feel better without the additional exercise effort. Leanness reveals detail. Looking stronger and bigger is not only about the amount of size your body has, but also has to do with definition and how visible your muscles are (especially if your goal is to look good on the beach).

Don't go to extremes though. Obsessing over body fat once you are around 9-12% for men and 16-21% percent for women is not always a healthy thing, either mentally or physically. If you want an aesthetic physique your goal should be on average below 15% all year round and maybe a bit closer to 10% in the holiday season if you want to look good on the beach.

A Couple of Words on the Advanced Phase

Going beyond the basic training level means that you will add a significant amount of stress on your body. The advanced level is not meant for everyone since a lot of discipline and compromise is required for it to work. Your life will be focused around your training program, which means that you will have to be seriously devoted to it. You will need to rethink a lot of your life's priorities and realize that this commitment will require you to focus a big part of your time in your training program and all the other extra aspects it's tied to (such as nutrition and rest). You will have to choose a goodnight sleep over staying up late with your friends. Your daily food should include a ton of protein. You will have to pass on that extra beer and you will probably have to get rid of all the useless habits (like watching TV) to find more free time to workout and rest. If you don't mind all these sacrifices and you want to take it a step further, you can move on to the advanced phase. This twelve month training program will bring you closer to your strength and physique's highest potential much faster. However, before you move on the advanced level, make sure you complete at least six months training with the basic level's program. You should also meet a couple requirements that I mention later on in this book.

Do This Before You Get Started

I want to talk to you a brief moment about the importance of taking a "before" photo once you decide to begin training. Why is this so important? Well think about it, this is something that won't cost you more than 20 seconds (just go next to a mirror and take a quick selfie with your phone).

Here is why you should to consider this:

- If you start losing motivation along the way you can look back at your "before" photo and remind yourself how you don't want to look like that ever again.

- As we mentioned previously, after your newbie gains, progress becomes slower. Therefore, if you have a monthly picture of your progress, it will make it easier to track your advancement.
- Get your picture posted on my website. Once you start seeing good results from your hard work, you can send me your before and after picture and I can upload it on my website. This is a cool way to show off to friends, girls or whoever. It's also a great reminder of what you accomplished. Plus it also helps me spread my message.
- Get personal training advice. Work hard, follow my plan and share your results with me and I'll give you a personal training consult through Skype for free!

Tips on Comparison Photography

If you want to take a proper before and after photo, here are some helpful tips:

1. For better contrast, choose a neutral background such as a white wall
2. Stand a few feet in front of the wall to minimize the sharpness of the shadow which may distract body outline. Note down your distance from the wall and the camera for next time.
3. It's better to have natural light as a light source. Ideally, the light source shouldn't be 90 degrees direct but in a slight angle (something like 70-80 degrees).

After all this, I am very excited that you have read this book so far because this is the part where things get interesting. Time to build HomeMade Muscle and become Strong & Lean without going to the Gym!

2

Warming Up

HERE IS A quote that you should engrain in your mind: "If you don't have enough time to warm-up, you don't have enough time to train." I always take my warm-up serious, since a proper warm-up has been proven to increase performance and reduce injuries probability. I hate watching results I have been building for months go down the drain just because I was too lazy to warm-up for ten minutes. In this eBook I include two warm-up methods, dynamic stretching and warm-up sets. For the beginners and the basic phase, dynamic stretching is enough. If you continue to the advanced phase, special warm-up sets are added after dynamic stretching.

Dynamic Stretching
A short definition of dynamic stretching would be - stretching as you are moving. Dynamic stretching is an active movement of your

body that brings forth a stretch but is not held statically in the end position.

When it comes to strength training, dynamic stretching and warm-up sets have been proven highly superior to "traditional" types of warm-up routines like jogging or static cycling. Traditional types like these don't really prepare you for the intensity and all the specific movement patterns of your workout. Think about it this way, during a strength workout, stress is applied to specific muscles, tendons, ligaments and joints; so how would static cycling or jogging prepare your upper body? For example, how would your shoulder joint be prepared for doing a simple push-up? The only positive effect cycling or jogging would have is by raising your temperature and warming up your legs. This is not bad of course, but it is also not enough.

Dynamic stretching on the other hand can prepare your body's connective tissues and muscles by performing targeted movements related to the movement patterns you will perform. More blood is pumped into the parts of the body you are about to train and their temperature rises. This will also increase your joints range of motion required to perform your exercises properly and injury-free. Once again, I am not saying that some jogging or cycling will hurt. For me, however, doing too much cardio before strength training takes my edge off. If you want to combine some traditional cardio exercise before dynamic stretching, five minutes to raise your body's temperature is enough. If you want to do more cardio for weight loss purposes, I would recommend doing it after your strength workout.

Go to my youtube channel at https://www.youtube.com/user/ HomeMadeMuscles and search for "Dynamic Stretching Routine")

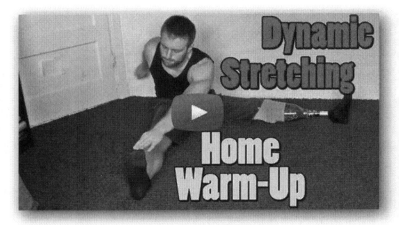

1. Neck rolls. Standing tall and relaxed, drop the chin close to your chest and gently roll the head toward one shoulder in a semicircular motion. Do 5 rolls in each direction (right and left shoulder) but be careful not to leave the head fall too far backwards. Make slow, big and fluid movements while keeping other muscles that aren't directly involved in the movement (like your shoulders) relaxed.

2. Shoulder rolls. The shoulder area is one of the most easily tensed areas in our bodies nowadays, due to bad postural habits, lifestyle and mental stress. Again standing tall and relaxed, start rotating your shoulders forwards in a big smooth, circular motion. Bring your shoulders up close to your ears and then back and down as low as possible. Repeat by doing the motion backwards this time. Start slow and increase the speed a bit after 15 seconds. Do two sets of 10 rolls with a 10-15 second rest in between.

3. Arm rotations. Start rotating your arms forward in a crossed position (right arm over left arm and try to alternate after every rotation). Keep your elbows slightly bent using a slow tempo. As you get used to the movements, increase the tempo a bit (as long as it feels comfortable). Do this for 20 seconds. Next rotate your arms forward, one at a time and each one for 15 seconds. Last, repeat all of this again but this time rotating your arms backwards.

4. Dynamic lat stretch. Stand with your feet shoulder width apart. Gently start to swing arms up and above your head and then back down all the way behind your body. Keep your elbows slightly bended during the movement. As you feel yourself loosening up and getting warmer, try to extend the arms further in each direction. Perform this exercise twice, for 20 seconds with a 10-15 second pause in between.

5. Dynamic chest stretch. Standing again with feet shoulder width apart, raise arms to chest height. Start swinging them across your chest and behind your body gradually increasing the speed a bit. Make sure you keep your arms close to chest height. Perform 10 repetitions twice with a pause of 10-15 seconds.

6. Dynamic shoulder stretch with elastic band. You can also find this exercise online called "Shoulder Dislocations" but I find that name a bit frightening. Don't worry, you aren't going to dislocate your shoulders (if you pay attention to my guidelines). This exercise is usually performed with special resistance bands. If you don't have one, just find a bicycle-wheel inner tube that you don't need any more. I'm sure there is one lying somewhere around your house. If not then you can buy a cheap one for just 2 dollars instead of spending 30 dollars for a regular resistance band. I actually prefer bicycle tubes because they have the ideal amount of elasticity, not to hard and not too soft. Many people use broomsticks as well but I highly recommend something with elasticity to make sure you don't injure your shoulders.

a) Start by holding the band about twice as wide as your shoulder width in front of you.
b) Start raising your arms up overhead. Be careful not to allow your shoulders to shrug upwards.
c) Bring the band all the way backwards, always making sure there is enough slack on it that allows you to do this movement without over-stressing your shoulders.

As you warm up you can slowly try to decrease the width of your grip on the band. The more you increase your flexibility in this exercise, the more you will be able to hold a narrower grip. Just make sure you always start wide enough and gradually decrease the width.

7. Alternating sitting toe touches (Windmill). This exercise will warm-up your back and open up your hamstrings without overstretching them. From a seated position, place your feet apart - about twice the distance of your shoulder width. Bend at the hips, and keep your spine straight and elongated (very important). Don't round your back! If you feel too much tension in your hamstrings bend your knees a little. From this position, perform the following:

a. Extend both arms out to your side, at shoulder height and
b. Rotate your trunk by bending a bit forward reaching with your arm towards the opposite toe.

c.   If you are not flexible, bend your knees enough in order to touch your toes (aim for tension not pain!)

d.   Alternate sides.

Note: If you do this exercise with bad form you can place unnecessary stress on your lower back so pay attention to proper form.

8. Chair Squats. This is more of a warm-up set but it's important in order to properly warm-up your legs. Find a chair that is not too tall; anything below knee height will do. Place a chair just behind you and stand in front of it. Place your feet shoulder-width apart or even a bit wider (whatever feels more comfortable) with your toes pointing a couple degrees outwards. Bend the knees and slowly squat towards the chair while keeping the weight on your heels (important). Avoid letting your knees surpass your toes. Sit on the chair for half a second and push up again through your heels, feeling at the same time your glutes push your body up. Fully extend the legs until you're back to a standing position. Repeat this for 3 sets of 5-20 repetitions.

Final Notes: Pay attention to the guidelines above for proper form and technique The general sensation we ought to have after completing an efficient warm-up should consist of the following basic points:

- Feeling our muscles stimulated enough and energized but not drained.
- Enough freedom of movement in our joints and muscles to perform all the exercises our basic program consists of.
- A rise in temperature enough to cause at least a mild perspiration.

It is far better to spend 15 minutes warming up every time, instead of training for months and watch all your results go down the drain, just because you skipped warm-up once and got injured.

3

Beginners

WHEN YOU'RE A beginner, you are far from your ultimate physical potential of strength and muscle growth. Your body doesn't know how to perform bodyweight exercises properly by activating neuromuscular pathways efficiently. This means that your body doesn't know yet how to combine strength and technique efficiently to use all the "horse power" it already has. The reason you improve a lot in the beginning of a strength training program is not only because your muscles grow bigger, but also because your nervous and muscular system learn to co-operate more effectively.

The more you perform an exercise, the more your neuromuscular system evolves and becomes more efficient at using every bit of neuronally-integrated muscle fiber that can facilitate this movement. Think of your neuromuscular efficiency as untapped strength you already have but cannot take advantage of. It's like having a fast car but not knowing how to drive yet. Focusing on proper technique in every exercise is essential in the beginners phase.

A beginner's ability to recover also improves. Recovery can be trainable to some extent, especially in the beginning.

Simply put, a beginner is someone for whom the stress applied during a single workout is enough to cause an adaptation until the next workout. This means that a beginner can become stronger in every single training session! This allows him to add repetitions or move to a more difficult progression in almost every workout during the first couple of weeks. After that, more reps or a more difficult progression can be performed about every two to three work outs. The end of the beginners phase is marked when the minimum progress of adding one rep or performing a more difficult progression every week ceases to happen. For people new to strength training this is usually somewhere between the second and third month.

The exercises that will be used as a criterion to the general guidelines above will be pull-ups and push-ups. Once you are able to perform at least 5 repetitions of pull-ups and push-ups with good form, then you are ready to move onto the advanced program. This doesn't mean that you shouldn't focus on improving your strength in the rest of the exercises, but these three particular exercises are the best criterion to test your pulling, squatting and pushing strength and to conclude with when you are ready to switch to the intermediate phase.

Beginners Program Structure

The beginner program is divided in two parts. Part A, which is the introductory program with the purpose to gradually introduce you to essential bodyweight concepts and exercises. It contains 4 basic exercises, each one focused on strengthening a primal movement pattern. The basic primal movement patterns are Pull, Push and Squat. To cover these you will do:

1. Pull-ups and Chin-ups as pulling pattern movements
2. Push-ups as a pushing pattern and
3. Lunges as a squatting pattern movement..

Supplementary exercises will also be included for your core. I say supplementary because no matter what exercise you do, bodyweight training always activates your core for stability and control (this is one of the cool benefits of bodyweight exercise).

- Your primal movement patterns are Pull, Push and squat

Phase A lasts three weeks. Because everybody differs in weight, height and strength, many people won't be able to perform the basic form of every exercise. Many people cannot do a pull-up once they get started. If you're one of them, don't let this overwhelm you. It's natural and I got your back. As mentioned previously, in the exercise menu you can find easier progressions for every movement. For example, even if you can't do regular push-ups, you can start with push-ups on your knees. Dips are not included in part A, but they will be added in Part B so that your shoulders can toughen up a bit first.

First week's goal is to experience a little soreness, but not so much that daily activities are impaired. Feeling some tenderness the next day, like for example below your armpits, in your chest, legs and glutes is to be expected. On the other hand, if lifting your glass of water is causing you pain, you could have gone a little easier on yourself...

Workout frequency in both phases is three times per week and one day of rest minimum is required between every session. You can train for example on - Monday, Wednesday and Friday or Tuesday - Thursday and Saturday. I like the first example because I prefer kicking back on the weekend. The program starts with pull-ups & chin-ups, doing 4 pulling sets in total. Combining these exercises two pulling variations in a workout builds immense upper body strength, especially in the arm and back areas.

Part A (3 Weeks)

	Exercises	Sets	Reps	Rest between sets	Rest between exercises
The Big Muscle Builders	1. Pull-Ups	2			
	2. Chin-Ups	2			
	3. Pistol Squats	4	5 -15	1 MINUTE	2 MINUTES
	4. Push-Ups	4			
Core	5. Leg Raises	3			
	6. Prone Cobra		3 sets of 40 - 60 seconds with 30 seconds rest		

Part B (5 -10 Weeks)

In every workout of the week there will be a difference in the exercise order. This way you focus once a week on each big muscle-building exercise, in the beginning of the program when your muscles are fully energized. Keep in mind that weighted lunges will always be placed in the middle of the program due to the fact that they are a lower body exercise. This way you give your upper body a bit more time to recover before continuing with the rest of the upper body exercises.

Workout #1

	Exercises	Sets	Reps	Rest between sets	Rest between exercises
The Big Muscle Builders	1. Pull-ups	2			
	2. Chin-Ups	2			
	3. Push-Ups	3			
	4. Pistol Squats	4	5 -15	1 MINUTE	2 MINUTES
	5. Dips	3			
Core	6. Leg Raises	3			
	7. Prone Cobra		3 sets of 40 - 60 seconds with 30 seconds rest		

Workout #2

	Exercise	Sets	Reps	Rest between sets	Rest between exercises
The Big Muscle Builders	1. Push-ups	3	5 -15	1 MINUTE	2 MINUTES
	2. Pull-ups	2			
	3. Chin-Ups	2			
	4. Pistol Squats	4			
	5. Dips	3			
Core	6. Leg Raises	3			
	7. Prone Cobra	3 sets of 40 - 60 seconds with 30 seconds rest			

(Workout 2 starts with dips. Make sure you
warm up your shoulders properly)

Workout #3

	Exercises	Sets	Reps	Rest between sets	Rest between exercises
The Big Muscle Builders	1. Dips	3	5 -15	1 MINUTE	2 MINUTES
	2. Pull-ups	2			
	3. Chin-Ups	2			
	4. Pistol Squats	4			
	5. Push-Ups	3			
Core	6. Leg Raises	3			
	7. Prone Cobra	3 sets of 40 - 60 seconds with 30 seconds rest			

The last workout of the week starts with Push-ups.

4

Basic

THE END OF a great era...The ending of the beginners phase is also the end of the "Newbie gains period." Anything you do related to strength training can produce some kind of muscle growth when you're a beginner. That's right - everything works! Even strength exercises such as running can cause some hypertrophy effect on your legs. Even doing 40 repetitions, which is far away from what the ideal rep range for strength and hypertrophy, can stimulate a significant amount of muscle growth when you're a novice. Still, this doesn't make all the crazy training programs out there valid (even though a lot of people get confused by this). Choosing an appropriate training method can extend the Newbie-Gains period as much as possible, so stick to a proper training program like HomeMade Muscle.

Some beginners might even respond better to a greater frequency than 3 workouts per week. This happens because they don't push themselves enough and are thus training with lower intensity than required. BUT it is important to establish a healthy training frequency from the beginning. This way it can be a frequency that will be maintained long-term and make your training program an inseparable part of your weekly routine. A three time per week training frequency in the beginning is enough to produce optimal muscle growth and strength while keeping you, at the same time, hungry enough for more. This will keep you motivated in the long run. Don't worry, there is more training volume coming later on if you are up to it!

After the newbie gains period starts to fade away, comes a critical time...this is when a big part of people gradually start to give up on their exercise program. Once plateaus start to hit their progress, they become discouraged. They might blame the training program and they're usually right. Most flashy training programs you stumble upon, whether you find them online or they were given to you by your neighborhood's gym, are only effective for beginners. Trainers get away with this because as we said, "everything works when you're new to strength exercise."

As your relationship with strength training deepens, you get to know your body better. You can now utilize your neuromuscular system more efficiently and push yourself closer to your strength potential. Although this is a great accomplishment, it also means that progress won't happen as often as it did in the beginning. It is now critical not to obsess on improvement from one workout to another. Sometimes progress won't even happen from week to week, but instead might take ten days, two or even three weeks towards the end of this phase. Don't worry, you are still on the right path. Be proud of your progress when it occurs and stick to your program.

Remember, nobody adds reps every week through eternity. The human species is a great adaptive organism but still, there's a limit to how fast you can adapt as you keep on improving.

Bodyweight athletes (that's you) who pass the beginners level, benefit from exposure to new movement patterns. This is why handstand push-ups and inverted rows are added at this point.

Basic Program Structure

The most demanding bodyweight exercises for the majority of people are Pull-ups, Handstand push-ups, and Dips. That is why the first three of them are placed in the beginning of one workout, once every week. This way, as mentioned previously in the book, you can hit them hard with your neuromuscular system fresh. As for weighted lunges, since they are a lower body exercise, they are placed in the middle of every routine so that you are not too drained and they can give your upper body a bit more time to recover before continuing with the rest of the upper body exercises

You will notice that there are some differences in the total amount of sets from day to day within the week. This is done for two reasons. Number one; there is always some extra volume in the first exercise of each workout (for the reasons mentioned in the previous paragraph). Number two; there is a decrease in sets of some other exercises that come later on in each training session. This is done in order to balance the total workload applied on pull and push movements.

The first workout of the week starts with pull-ups & chin-ups doing 6 sets in total. Combining these exercises together builds immense upper body strength, especially in the arm and back department. Because these two exercises have very similar movement patterns, they will be considered to be part of the same exercise - exercise one.

Workout #1

	Exercise	Sets	Reps	Rest between sets	Rest between exercises
Big Muscle Builders	1. A. Pull-ups	3			
	B. Chin-ups	2			
	2. Handstand Push-ups	3			
	3. Pistol Squats	4	5-15	1 MINUTE	2 MINUTES
	4. Dips	3			
	5. Inverted Rows	2			
	6. Push-ups	3			
Core	7. Leg Raises	3			
	8. Prone Cobra	3 sets of 40 - 60 seconds with 30 seconds rest			

Average time to complete Workout: 1 hour

Workout 2 starts with handstand push-ups. Remember, handstand push-ups take a while to accomplish. Once you are able to perform this highly intense exercise, make sure you thoroughly warm up your shoulders. Adding some handstands on a wall and two sets of pike push-ups to your warm up sets before doing the exercise is a good idea.

Workout #2

	Exercise		Sets	Reps	Rest between sets	Rest between exercises
Big Muscle Builders	1.	Pike Push-ups	4			
	2.	A. Pull-ups	2			
		B. Chin-ups	2	5 -15	1 MINUTE	2 MINUTES
	3.	Pistol Squats	4			
	4.	Push-ups	2			
	5.	Inverted Rows	3			
	6.	Dips	3			
Core	7.	Leg Raises	3			
	8.	Prone Cobra		3 sets of 40 - 60 seconds with 30 seconds rest		

Average time to complete Workout: 1 hour

The last workout of the week starts with dips which are one of the best bodyweight exercises for the chest. This is the last day of the week, so warm-up well and don't be afraid to push yourself. There will be plenty of time to recover during the next two resting days.

Workout #3

	Exercises	Sets	Reps	Rest between sets	Rest between exercises
	1. Dips	4			
	2. A. Pull-ups	2			
	B. Chin-ups	2			
Big Muscle Builders	3. Pistol Squats	4	5 - 15	1 MINUTE	2 MINUTES
	4. Pike push-ups	3			
	5. Inverted Rows	3			
	6. Push-ups	2			
Core	7. Leg Raises	3			
	8. Prone Cobra	3 sets of 40 - 60 seconds with 30 seconds rest			

Average time to complete Workout: 1 hour

5

Advanced

FOR THOSE OF you willing to move on to the advanced level, I highly recommend a complete week off. Give your joints and tendons a break to recover properly.

As I mentioned previously, the advanced phase is for serious bodyweight athletes. If you decide to go forward on this challenging path, I salute you and I promise I am going to be next to you the entire way. Anytime you need me, just e-mail me at homemademusclemail@gmail.com and add "advanced level" in the subject area. That being said, it's time for some serious work so let's get started...

The advanced training level consists of a twelve-month plan which is divided in main three phases. Phase one lasts three months; phase two and three both last four months. There is also a transitional week in the beginning to ease into the program. I highly recommend this if you took some time off after completing the Basic Program or if you are an experienced bodyweight athlete and skipped the first two programs (Beginner's & Basic). To perfect this twelve month program, I went through a lot of trial and error. For an entire year, I experimented and trained 10-15 training hours per week to perfect it. In the end I looked, felt and became stronger then I ever was. And So will you! In fact, you will be even better off than I was since you don't have to go through my mistakes now that the program is perfected.

Increasing Training Frequency

As you remember training frequency is important and you should train using whole-body workouts at least three times per week when it comes to bodyweight exercise for optimum progress. If done properly, you can increase frequency by lowering a bit of your intensity. Training more frequently will benefit you at this point because you will improve your neuromuscular efficiency faster this way. As we discussed in strength basics - factors like coordination, balance and kinesthetic awareness - are part of performing complex exercises such as one arm push-ups and handstand push-ups. Increased training frequency can help you a lot during this phase of your development as a bodyweight athlete.

Unless you are blessed with the genetics of a talented gymnast, frequency is more important than intensity at this point. This does not mean that you will train lightly. It just means that you will not be going to failure on low intensity days. Used in a proper organized training program, high frequency will make you stronger, faster and bigger.

Simply said: More frequency minus a bit intensity = more strength = more gains

Preliminaries (IMPORTANT)

Besides training with the basic program for at least six months, I have three basic prerequisites you should meet in order to make sure you are ready for the Advanced Phase, as follows:

1. Pull-ups - 10 clean reps (chest to bar)
2. Weighted lunges - 10 clean reps with a 20kg weighted back-pack (45 lbs)
3. Handstand push-ups - 5 clean reps (head slightly touching the floor)

If you cannot perform these exercises with good form just yet, stick to the Basic Program for a while longer.

6 The Number of the Beast

If you want to become a bodyweight beast, this is the exact number of exercises you are going to need to focus on in the basic part of every training session - six basic movements. While developing this program, I only had one thing on my mind - how to get the best out of the minimum. Thinking in terms of anatomy and kinesiology, these were also the best bodyweight exercises to strengthen the body to its greatest potential while keeping it in balance.

<u>This is how the main part of your workout should look by the end of the year:</u>

1. Handstand Push-ups
2. Weighted Lunges

3. Pull-ups (chest to bar)
4. One arm-push-ups
5. Dragon Flags
6. One arm dead hangs

Don't worry if you're not yet at the point were you can do one-arm push-ups and dragon flags. Neither could I when I started working on this program. Follow this program to the letter, lose the extra weight that is weighing you down and by the end of the year you will be a mean one arm push-up machine training abs Bruce Lee style.

One-Arm Deadhangs

A new exercise that is added in this level is Dead-hangs. Forearms and grip strength are quite neglected in most of today's training programs. If you are a beginner, then just doing simple pull-ups is enough for developing this area. But if you go past the point of a beginner, you will need to include specialized training in order to further develop these muscles. It might surprise you how difficult it can be to just hang with one arm on a pull up bar. Think about it; if you compare it to a simple two-arm dead-hang, which you are used to doing, you are now adding twice the intensity.

Grip Strength Importance: Unless you're genetically gifted with thick forearms, they can be quite resistant to growth. A pair of muscular forearms is quite impressive visually but that is not the only reason you should strengthen them. Grip strength adds strength to all pulling exercises, it can help you overcome pull-up plateaus, and in general they allow better stability and control during most pulling related bodyweight exercises. The main reason this happens can be described by the principle of "Irradiation." This principle states that you can contract a muscle harder if you also contract the muscles surrounding it.

<u>If this all sounds a little weird, try the following experiment:</u>

1. Try flexing your bicep as hard as possible without making a fist.

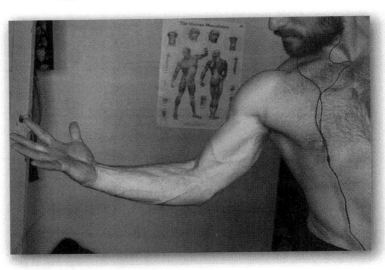

2. Now try to flex your bicep as hard as possible while making a fist and squeezing it really tight.

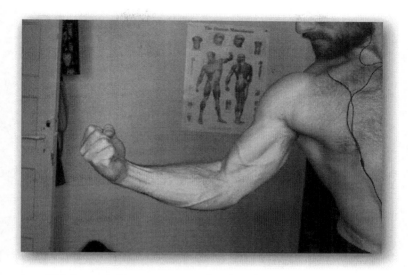

Didn't your bicep contract harder the second time? Grip strength is also extremely important if your goal is to achieve a one-arm pull-up in the future.

Why Dead-hangs?

I tried several ways to strengthen my forearms during 2013, I even bought those 70's grippers. Well...that was a big waste of money. Served me right for making such a stupid compulsive purchase, I could easily have avoided just by using my brain for ten seconds. I mean seriously, how is sitting in front of the TV and squeezing these grippers a couple of hundred times a day, going to improve your grip strength? Also, how is it going to add functional strength to your training program? Our forearms need progressive overload and a rep range of 1-15 repetitions or (if you are using isometrics) a total time under tension of 5-60 seconds in order to get stronger, just like most of the muscles in our body. What can be more functional in developing grip strength than hanging on something? When it comes to strength training, generally the simplest solution is the most effective.

Forearm Recovery

In order to aid your recovery a bit more, it is a good idea to add some soft tissue work on your forearms while developing them. Find a ball about the size of a tennis ball but a bit harder. Like a lacrosse ball, a golf ball or a baseball. Place a towel on the table (so that it's less slippery) and apply pressure on your forearms by rolling them on the ball against the table.

After your soft tissue work, you can add a simple stretch for your fingers. Just put your fingers on the edge of a table and softly press so that they extend. Once finished, do the same thing with your thumbs. Two or three sets of twenty seconds is enough.. More on how to build those Popeye forearms in the exercise menu.

Warming Up

Another parameter that changes in this phase is your warm up. You are now at a point that your body knows how to tap into your body's ultimate horse power. This also means that you need to warm up even more efficiently to avoid stressing your joints and ligaments. In fact, in this training level, the warm up is half the workout. Yes, you read that correct, half the workout!

"The warm up is half the workout"

Inverted rows, push-ups, bilateral (two legged) squats and prone cobras are now part of your warm up. You body has now matured enough to use easy-sets (low intensity) of these exercises in order to warm up and prepare yourself for the remainder of the program. Inverted Rows will prepare you for pulling movements. Push-ups will prepare your wrists, elbows & shoulders for pushing movements. Bilateral squats will warm up your legs and prone cobras will warm up the whole back chain all the way up from your head, through your upper and lower back, and down to your glutes and hamstrings. Warming up this way will also add a little more "easy strength to the bank" without exhausting you for the rest of the program.

1. Start your warm up with our dynamic stretching routine.
2. Rest for 30-60 seconds and move on to easy sets.

Easy Sets
Sensation: While doing these sets you are not supposed to be experiencing any great amount of fatigue. A mild "pump" to get some blood flowing in your muscles is what you're aiming for.
Warm up sets order:

1. Inverted rows
2. Push-ups
3. Bodyweight squats
4. Prone cobra

Sets and Rest: These exercises are going to be performed in a form of circuit training. After each exercise rest briefly (5-10 seconds max) and move on. Once you are finished with one round of all four exercises, rest for ninety seconds and repeat. You are going to complete a total of two to three rounds. Two rounds are enough if you are working out in a warm environment and if you've been awake for more than six hours. Three rounds are required if you train early in the morning and/or in cold environments.

Reps: The number of reps should be about half the reps you would need to do, in order to come close to failure in an exercise by doing 3 sets with one minute rest in between. If you have completed the basic level training, then you now that exact number but let's see an example just to be sure. If you would do three sets of 15 push-ups with one minute rest in between in order to come close to failure, then your warm up sets should consist of 7-8 repetitions. Remember to balance this number with the sensation described above. Feel free to add or reduce a few of reps to get the right feeling.

Introduction Part (1 Week)

The first week is meant to ease you into the program and get you accustomed with the main philosophy and purpose. It consists of three training sessions with each training session having at least one day of rest in between. There are two types of workouts: Workout A and Workout B, which will also be included in the Advanced Phases. The main difference between workout A and B is the order of the exercises (for the same reasons mentioned in previous chapters). Specifically, workout A begins with Handstand Push-ups whereas workout B starts with Pull-ups. These two exercises are the two basic cornerstones of HomeMade Muscle and that is why it is crucial that you perform them in the beginning of your workout.

Rule #1 of the Advanced Program - Never go until failure on workouts A & B.

Intensity should not be very high in workouts A & B in order for this program to work. Remember increasing frequency needs to occur strategically. All of your sets should be performed with perfect form. Use perfect technique in every set and every rep!

- Have good control over your body in every single rep; observe and focus on muscle contraction.
- Don't just pull or push yourself up - contract your muscles consciously.
- Feel the floor or the bar in every movement, don't just hang or depend on them.
- Be aware not only of the whole movement, but also of the movement as a whole.

Important Note: Until this point you have just been doing reps. *"I now want you to experience conscious movement against gravity".*

Once you get to the point where you feel that your next rep might not be performed with perfect form or might fail - stop. If you miscalculate and you come close to failure, simply quit the rep at that point instantly. You will learn to do this more efficiently over time.

Here is an example with pull-ups to make this even clearer. Let's say you are doing 3 sets of 10 repetitions. Your first set should be relatively easy. In the second set, somewhere after 6-7 reps you should be starting to feel quite heavy. In set number three your last 3 reps should be tough enough so that you have to put a more effort in them, but not that tough that you break form. All three sets should be done with outstanding form.

Transitional week						
Monday	Tuesday	Wednesday	Thursday	Friday	Saturday	Sunday
Workout A	Rest	Workout B	Rest	Workout A	Rest	

Workout A				
Exercise	Repetitions	Sets	Rest between sets	Rest between exercises
1. Handstand push-ups	5 -15	3	75 seconds	1 -2 minutes
2. Pistol Squats				
3. Pull-ups				
4. Push-ups (aim for one arm push-ups)				
5. Leg Raises (aim for Dragon Flags)				
6. One-arm Dead Hangs	Start with 3-5 "			

Now that you have reached the Advanced Training Level, you should be getting closer to exercises like one arm push-ups and dragon flags. Work on the progressions and variations of these exercises and don't worry if you still feel far from achieving these. Using the Advanced Level Training Program will get you there before you know it. All you need is patience and consistency.

Workout B				
Exercise	Repetitions	Sets	Rest between sets	Rest between exercises
1. Pull-ups	5 -12	3	75 seconds	1 -2 minutes
2.Pistol Squats				
3.Handstand push-ups				
4.Push-ups (aim for one-arm push-ups)				
5.Leg Raises (Dragon Flags)				
6. One-arm Dead Hangs	Start with 3-5"			

Phase 1 (3 months)

Phase 1 lasts three months and consists of four training sessions per week. You will start your week with two back-to-back training days followed by one day off. That means you will be doing Workout A on day one and Workout B on day two. After resting on day three, you will perform again Workout A on day four and Workout B on day five. Day six and day seven are resting days.

Due to the increased training frequency, it is possible that you will feel "heavy" the first twenty days of Phase 1. Don't worry if this happens. Once you get past these days and have the low volume training week I prescribe, your body will adapt and your performance will go up again. This is how your weekly plan will look (assuming that you begin your training week on Mondays).

Weekly Schedule						
Monday	Tuesday	Wednesday	Thursday	Friday	Saturday	Sunday
Workout A	Workout B	Rest	Workout A	Workout B	Rest	

Workout A				
Exercise	Repetitions	Sets	Rest between sets	Rest between exercises
1. Pull-ups	5-12	3		
2. Pistol Squats	5 -15	4		
3. Handstand push-ups				
4. Push-ups (aim for one-arm push-ups)	5-12	3	75 seconds	1 -2 minutes
5. Leg raises (Dragon Flags)	5 - 15	3		
6. One-arm Dead Hangs	Start with 5-10"	3		

Workout B				
Exercise	Repetitions	Sets	Rest between sets	Rest between exercises
1. Pull-ups	5-12	3		
2. Pistol Squats	5 -20	4		
3. Handstand push-ups				
4. Push-ups (aim for one-arm push-ups)	5-12	3	75 seconds	1 -2 minutes
5. Leg Raises (Dragon Flags)	5-8	3		
6. One-arm Dead Hangs	Start with 5-10"	3		

Low Volume Week

From now on every time you complete four weeks of continuous training you will have a low volume training week as described below. This will allow your neuromuscular system to recover properly.

Low volume training Week (once every 4 weeks)						
Monday	Tuesday	Wednesday	Thursday	Friday	Saturday	Sunday
Workout A	Rest	Workout B	Rest	Workout A	Rest	

Rule #2 of the Advanced Program - Have a low volume training week every four weeks.

Phase 2 (4 months)

Before moving on to Phase 2, instead of having a low volume training week, take a whole week off. Trust me, you are going to need it for the next phase. Do not worry, nobody's physique and strength fell apart from taking a single week off once every couple of months. On the other hand, there are many people out there who achieved a great physique and amazing strength levels but did not last very long due to problems such as bad shoulders, elbow pain or repetitive knee injuries. If you worry about issues like gaining weight, etc., just stay active during this week by doing low intensity cardio activities. Go for a one-hour long walk in the morning or a jog for thirty minutes, three times per week and you'll be fine.

Rule #3 of the Advanced Program - Take a week off whenever you switch from one phase to another.

Taking one week off replenishes muscle glycogen storage, helps you avoid overuse injuries and lets your muscles and especially the nervous system, recover properly. There might be a slight feeling of strength loss when you get back to your program but don't worry. You'll be back on track after two workout sessions.

To avoid extreme muscle soreness, go easy on your first workout after your whole week off. Otherwise, too much soreness will get in the way later on.

Rule #4 of the Advanced Program - Always go easy on your first workout after a whole week off.

Phase 2 lasts four months and consists of five training sessions per week. You will start your week with two back-to-back training days followed by a day off. That means you will be doing Workout A on day one and Workout B on day two. After resting on day three, you will repeat the same on day four and day five. On day six you will perform Workout C and on day seven you will rest again. Once again, due to the increased training frequency, it is possible that you will feel "heavy" the first three to four weeks of Phase 2. Once you get past these weeks and have a low volume training week, your body will adapt and your performance will go up again. This is how your weekly plan will look:

Weekly Schedule						
Monday	Tuesday	Wednesday	Thursday	Friday	Saturday	Sunday
Workout A	Workout B	Rest	Workout A	Workout B	Workout C	Rest

(Workouts A and B are the same as in Phase 1)

Workout C - Rest/Pause technique

In Workout C you will be using a popular strength developing technique called Rest/Pause. The Rest/Pause technique became popular by a famous 1960's power lifter named Jim Williams. In his early life big Jim had been involved in some criminal activity and was sentenced to ten years in prison. Due to the limited equipment available in the prison, this technique helped him train hard without using a lot of weight.

What you need to know about the Rest/Pause technique

Rest/Pause training divides your training set with a brief resting period of 15 seconds that allows you to do a couple more reps. For example, let's say you can perform three sets of ten pull-ups with about a minute of rest between each set. Using the Rest/Pause technique, once you are finished with ten repetitions, you rest for 15 seconds and add two to three more reps. After that, you rest and repeat 2 more sets.

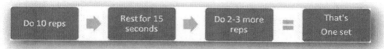

| Do 10 reps | Rest for 15 seconds | Do 2-3 more reps | That's One set |

This technique will give you a great muscle pump and will add extra (metabolic) stress to your muscles. It is believed that the effects of metabolic stress increases muscle fiber recruitment and enhances the growth potential of the muscle as a whole. Although exercise scientists (such as hypertrophy expert Brad Schoenfield) are still researching this, it has been one of the classic secret tools bodybuilders use to get big since the rise of their sport. Besides that, it also makes your workouts more challenging and motivational! Because Rest/Pause sets are quite demanding, you will only focus on two exercises. These are our favorite Handstand push-ups and Pull-ups.

Note: Never go to failure in handstand push-ups. Shoulders need a lot of work and time to get used to this exercise until you can go hard at it without risking injury. Pull-ups on the other hand can take more of a beating so feel free to go all in with this exercise on Workout C.

Program C - Rest/Pause		
Exercise	Sets and Reps	Rest
1.Handstand push ups	a) Begin with a set of the same reps you performed in training A.	
	b) Once you complete the reps, rest 15 seconds and add 2-3 more reps. That was one whole rest/pause set.	• Between each set: 2 min
2.Pull ups		• From exercise to exercise: 4 min
	c) Do three sets in total.	

Don' forget your low volume training week

Phase 3 (4 months)

Again, before moving on to this next Phase take a whole week off followed by the transition week. Phase 3, just like Phase 2, consists of five training sessions per week.

Low volume training Week (once every 4 weeks)						
Monday	Tuesday	Wednesday	Thursday	Friday	Saturday	Sunday
Workout A	Rest	Workout B	Rest	Workout A	Rest	

(Workouts A and B remain the same as in Phase 1 & 2)

Workout C - Reversed Pyramid

The reason this workout is called the "Reversed Pyramid" is because of the way the repetitions are structured. You begin your first set by doing 50% of the total repetitions you would do on Workout A or B. After that, you rest one minute and add one more rep. Continue doing this until you fail to add another rep. Again, because this program is quite tough, you are only going to do two exercises - Handstand push-ups and Giant pull-ups.

If this seems a bit complicated, let's have a look at an **example** with pull-ups. Let's say that the amount of pull-ups you do on a regular workout such as Workout B is eight. This is how your reversed pull-up pyramid will look:

- 1st Set: Do 4 reps (50%) and rest for one minute.
- 2nd set: Do 5 reps and rest for one minute.
- 3rd set: Do 6 reps and rest for one minute etc

Do this until your reach the first set where you fail to add another rep with perfect form.

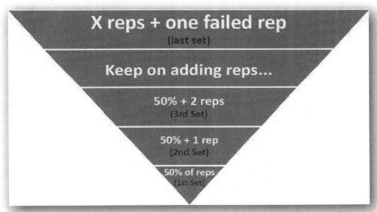

Workout C - Reversed Pyramid		
Exercise	Sets and Reps	Rest
1.Handstand push ups	• Start with 50% of the total reps you perform in Workout A. • After every set add one repetition until you reach a set you cannot complete.	• In the beginning rest **one minute** after every set. • When you feel you are approaching your last set rest **90 seconds**
1.Giant pull ups	• Start with 50% of the total reps you perform in 3 sets in Workout B. • After every set, add one repetition until you reach a set you cannot complete.	

Low Volume Week

Just as in Phase 1 and 2, every time you complete 4 weeks of continuous training you will add a low volume training week as described below.

Basic Rules of the Advanced Phase:

1. Never go until failure on Workouts A & B.
2. Have a low volume training week every 4 weeks.
3. Take a week off whenever you switch from one phase to another
4. Always go easy on your first workout after a whole week off.

Part 4

Nutrition

ALL DIETS WORK, until they don't. Get started on any diet plan and I guarantee you that you will lose some weight or feel better in the beginning. Also, some diets work good for some people but not so good for others. After extensively studying nutrition, I understand that it can be a frustrating subject to research. Everyday new diets arise, nutrition specialists and the even the USDA change their opinions on what is healthy or not. And the number of obese people continues to rise... Nowadays, statistics show that even though more people are on more diets than ever before, we are also fatter than ever.

1

Lost in diet land

WHEN I FIRST began my healthy-eating journey, I quickly became a victim of countless fad diets. As Denise Minger says in her great book - Death by Food Pyramid, "*I had fallen under the spell that seduces health voyagers; the power of unsubstantiated anecdote and well-posed before and after pictures.*"

Since I wasn't the best critical thinker at the time, I just read all the popular diet books available on Amazon. The criteria I used to judge them was probably identical with everybody else; I just paid attention to the shinny 5-star reviews, the fancy PhD titles next to the authors names and all the "scientific" studies quoted in them (which I never cared to examine). To my defense, the educational system I grew up in (as probably most educational systems) never taught me critical thinking skills. The Sports Science University I graduated from had a course on nutrition (taught by a suspiciously overweight nutrition professor) and focused primarily on the typical food pyramid, which didn't seem to work, either for me or the rest of the world.

The Truth About Weight Loss.

If you only care about controlling your weight, then the solution is simple (although not practical). If you're a healthy individual, losing weight is strictly a matter of calories in and calories out. Your body burns a specific amount of calories every day, which you can easily calculate if you go online. If you are not familiar with calorie calcula-tors, just Google something like "free daily calorie intake calculator" and you will find a ton of free calorie calculators. After that, it is just a matter of counting your calories every day (although this is a pain in the ass). If you want to lose weight you have to be on a caloric deficit and if you want to gain weight, you have to be on a caloric surplus. Some of you reading this might be quite skeptical; I also was a couple of years ago.

A nutritionist from the University of Kansas named Mark Haub performed the following experiment. He followed a hypocaloric diet based on 70% junk food such as Doritos, Oreos, cereals based on sugar and other foods with "empty calories." The rest of his calories came from some veggies, a protein supplement and a multivitamin. Results after 10 weeks? He lost 27 pounds and his blood work improved! Of course we don't know what the long term health effects of that diet would be and neither I nor Mark Haub think it would be a healthy dietary approach in the long run. The professor himself obviously doesn't recommend this diet to anyone and the reason he did this experiment was to prove that a diet doesn't have to be 100% clean in order to be healthy as many nutritional and fitness gurus out there suggest.

Special Diets

The only diets supported by solid scientific evidence that might have a slight benefit over the general rule of caloric intake, are high protein diets. High protein diets have a slight benefit, mainly due to the fact that protein is a macronutrient that has a greater thermogenic effect on your body. This means that in comparison with fat and carbs, your body uses more energy in order to break down protein (or what is also called protein catabolism, which is the process of your body dissolving protein macromolecules into amino acids and other simple derivative compounds to serve all kinds of functions in your body).

Another hot topic currently is fasting related diets such as Intermittent Fasting. Some say that they might have a small metabolic advantage mainly due to the hormonal manipulation that occurs from the fasting periods these diets have. Still there is no solid scientific evidence to support something like this, since at the end of the day the human body tends to balance out most of these hormonal fluctuations.

The main point here is that no matter what diet you choose, if your daily calories overextend your daily caloric needs, you will, without a doubt, gain weight after a certain point. Of course the media, doctors, and other health specialists who want to promote their new "groundbreaking" diet books and other products, will try to mislead you. When you are trying to lose weight, the truth is as simple as doing some calorie-math. No matter what you hear, keep in mind that all the serious and unbiased scientific research backs this up.

How Diets Trick You Into Losing Weight

Diets help you lose weight by tricking you into eating less. While that might not sound bad, it can lead to unhealthy eating behaviors in the long run. For example, let's take Paleo diet. Paleo cuts out most carbs, sugar and processed food, which means that you can only eat food categories like meat, nuts and fruits. One problem with this diet approach is that it's really difficult to fill all your caloric needs based on these few food categories - trust me I've tried! No wonder people "miraculously" lose weight on Paleo. If you're overweight, it can work for a long time but at some point you will end up starved. Another trick Paleo and other diets use is encouraging you to eat more protein. Protein has shown to be the most satiating macronutrient. This means that eating high-protein foods helps you feel full for longer periods of time, which again helps you eat less.

Let's also examine an opposite diet like veganism. Vegan diets help a lot of people lose weight because they exclude two other major food categories, meat & dairy. At the same time, they also encourage you to eat more fiber, water and total food volume, which is again a good strategy to lose weight and to feel better! There is nothing wrong with strategies that help you eat less and healthier of course.

Eating enough protein and a lot of vitamin and mineral dense foods is important. However, what bothers me is when diet-book authors use these strategies secretly, making false claims. Making you falsely thing that the foods you are excluding from your diet are what is making you overweight and unhealthy. This can lead to very unhealthy eating behaviors in the long run.

Why Do Diets Make You Feel Better?

Another thing that confused me when experimenting with a few diets is that I was experiencing a big energy boost. There were periods, especially in the beginning, when I was eating less and even sleeping less, yet I felt unstoppable. I was a lean mean exercise machine! As I learned later, the reason this occurs is not due to the magic powers of the diet. Instead it was due to elevated Catecholamines; also known as the "flight or fight response" hormones. Adrenaline (epinephrine), noradrenaline (norepinephrine) and dopamine can increase your heart rate, blood pressure, breathing rate, muscle strength, mental alertness and even produce a feeling of euphoria. Catecholamines are often released into the bloodstream due to stress or fright and prepare the body for the "fight-or-flight" response. Mystery solved. Although I love the energy surplus I experience on a hypocaloric diet, unfortunately you can't keep on losing weight for ever.

2

Breakfast:
Not the most important meal of the day

For SOME OF you who stay current with the latest updates in nutrition, this won't be anything new to you. For others, it may even sound crazy... "But I have been told all my life by parents, doctors and TV commercials that breakfast is this most important meal of the day, what the hell are you talking about?!" you will think.

The Shocking Truth Behind Cereal
The common notion is that when you haven't eaten anything for a whole night, once your body wakes up, it immediately needs a meal rich in carbs to have energy for the rest of the day's mental and physical tasks. Not eating breakfast will damage your metabolism, make you fat, decrease your energy, and maybe cause world war 3 - who knows! The truth is simple, think about it from an evolutionary point. Did our hunter and gatherer ancestors who lived in the wild

for hundreds and thousands of years have food available to them the moment they woke up? The answer is no, of course. They had to hunt or at least go out and wander around in the wild to gather their food. Prepackaged and ready to eat breakfast cereals began with the American temperance movement in the 19th century. In a species that is around earth for a hundreds & thousands of years, that's quite a small segment of time. We might not live as hunters and gatherers anymore but the modern lifestyle which considers breakfast the most important meal of the day began as a habit that was forced upon us in the USA by people like John Harvey Kellogg.

Surprisingly, cereal wasn't originally a cynical marketing ploy to sell sugar to children if that was your original thought.

In the 1830s, the Reverend Sylvester Graham preached the virtues of a vegetarian diet to his congregation, and in particular the importance of whole-meal flour. "Meat-eating," he said, "excited the carnal passions." After that, the Seventh-Day Adventists John Harvey Kellogg took up the mission. He set about devising cures for what he believed were the common ills of the day; in particular constipation and masturbation (wtf right?). In Kellogg's mind, the two were closely linked. Kellogg experimented in the sanitarium kitchen to produce an easily digested form of cereal.

That's right; breakfast cereal was a cynical marketing ploy by religious fundamentalists to destroy your sex drive! Isn't that just dandy!?

Reality and Science Behind Breakfast.

In typical healthy individuals cortisol levels peak every morning after a good night sleep for about an hour to ninety minutes after you wake up. This normal spike of cortisol helps break down body fat by increasing the release of fatty acids for fuel. Some of you might ask yourselves, "won't Cortisol also break down muscle?" Here is where growth hormone comes to the rescue. Another thing that happens in the morning is the release of a hormone called Ghrelin. Besides making you feel hungry, Ghrelin also stimulates the release of Growth Hormone which also stimulates fat burn and doesn't allow your body to burn muscle tissue just by abstaining from food for half a day. When you start consuming big sugary bowls of cereal and in general foods rich in carbs in the morning, you spike up your insulin which shuts downs the production of all the hormones associated with fat burn I mentioned above. I'm not trying to say anything out of the norm here, all I want to say is that when you start eating your body stops burning fat and starts burning food (duuh).

Most people, once they get used to it, function a lot better without breakfast. They also notice better energy levels. The reason for this is that after having fasted for about 8-10 hours (while sleeping), when you wake up your body turns on your sympathetic nervous system, which is basically your "fight or flight" mode. When you eat a breakfast rich in carbs, insulin production increases and you over-stimulate your opposite-parasympathetic mode, which in simple words means you start feeling lazy and sleepy. That's the main reason most people feel sleepy in the morning hours at work and need a liter of coffee to get through these "heavy" hours.

Still some people (especially women) don't function well when skipping breakfast. If that's the case with you, try starting your day with a meal high in protein like an omelet. Keep in mind that even though I'm an advocate of skipping breakfast, it doesn't mean I don't enjoy Sunday morning pancakes every now and then. Once you have reached your ideal weight, your diet can become quite flexible if you follow some basic rules we will talk about later on.

Special Weight Loss Diets – What Works For Me

Let's face it...No matter how many tips you find on dieting and no matter what strategies you use, if you want to lose a lot of weight you will experience some moments of hunger. Still, it's not the worst thing that could happen to you. The human spirit has gone through some really hard situations in the past, people have gone through war, slavery, torture and so much more. So man-up and stop looking for excuses! Set your weight goals and make it clear to yourself that until then, you will be disciplined.

We have established that counting calories is the most efficient way to lose weight, yet it's also not the most practical one. Having a general idea of how many calories you are eating and being able to calculate calories of the typical foods you eat on a daily basis can be very helpful. Foods like eggs, oatmeal, brown bread, fruits and nuts are typical things I eat on a daily basis. Due to this, I know how many calories are in these foods which helps me have a general idea of my daily caloric intake.

Because I tend to get lazy though on counting calories for every single meal I have, I don't obsess over calorie counting and I just focus on some basic eating strategies when I want to lose some weight. What I do is I focus on reducing carbs, junk food and only allow myself to eat in a specific time window. A method that helps a lot with the programming of the latter is Intermittent fasting.

3

Intermittent Fasting &
The myth of frequent meals

Most of you have heard that eating small frequent meals speeds up your metabolism and does all kinds of magical things. The truth is that this is also just a myth which science once again has disproven. We have become so brainwashed today when it comes to food, that we are afraid of staying unfed for even a couple of hours. We think that it will screw up our metabolism or burn all our muscles. Once again, I was also a victim of this eating myth until I read books like Orie Hofmekler's book "The Warrior Diet," Jason Ferrugia's "The Renegade Diet" and "Eat Stop Eat" by Brad Pilon. These books changed my perspective on nutrition and broadened my research on fasting diets.

The human body is an amazing organic machine and wouldn't have survived hundreds of thousands of years in the wild if it suffered such consequences when it stayed unfed for as little as 16 hours. Do you think your cavemen ancestors had a fridge in his cave where they could go and have a snack whenever they felt they had the "munchies"?

I know fasting may sound a bit scary at first if you are not familiar with this diet technique, however don't be afraid... You don't have to wander around the desert of Jerusalem for 40 days like Jesus in order to fast. Intermittent fasting **(IF)** divides your daily eating schedule into 2 phases: 1) a fasting phase; and 2) an eating phase. The only important thing to watch when you are doing intermittent fasting is to remain hydrated during the fasting phase. If you think about it, we all fast intermittently at night when we sleep. The only thing that changes usually in IF is that you fast for a couple of hours more after you wake up. Just think of IF as simply skipping breakfast in the beginning, it will make the whole process a lot easier.

In order to fast intermittently, you eat your last meal 3-4 hours before you go to bed. I personally eat my last meal around 7 - 8pm since I go to sleep at 11pm. After fasting for 16 hours you can have your first meal the next day around 11am - 12pm. I try not to go beyond 16 hours, otherwise I don't have enough time to fulfill my caloric needs without compromising my energy levels by having to eat huge meals during the rest of day.

During the fasting phase (8pm – 12 noon the next day) I always make sure to stay hydrated, especially in the morning hours and during my workout, since I train in a fasted state. Other than water, you can also have coffee and tea. If you want to add sugar to your coffee or tea, avoid adding more than one teaspoon.

As with every diet, there is going to be a brief adaptation phase in the beginning for everyone. But generally after 3-7 days most people start noticing the benefits of this eating-style. Improved energy levels, mental clarity (especially in the morning fasted hours) and improved productivity in mental and physical activities are some common benefits people experience (including me). If you find it too difficult to begin fasting for 16 hours, you can start progressively with 12 hours and add one hour every one or two days until you reach 16 hours.

Personally, giving my body a break from eating, helps me function better. This is noticeable especially during the fasting phase in which I experience increased energy levels and I can also concentrate more effectively on my everyday's tasks. One of the reasons this happens as believed by authors of fasting diets, is that your body gets a break from digesting food all the time and your nervous system can focus more on the rest of your body's voluntary (e.g. concentration) and involuntary (e.g. energy levels and liver detoxification) tasks.

Basic Guidelines of IF:

- Eat a fulfilling meal 3-4 hours before bed time;
- After that, fast for 16 hours (calorie-free liquids are allowed)
- Once you break your fast, you have an 8-hour window to consume the amount of calories, micro and micronutrients your body requires.
- Some of the people I wouldn't recommend fasting, are the following:
- Kids whose bodies are still developing;
- Special groups of population with health issues (this goes for any advice in this book of course)

- People with high metabolic rates who are trying to build muscle or highly competitive athletes who need big amounts of calories to sustain their weight
- People, especially women, who find they don't feel very well after a week of this fasting routine.

Training in a Fasted State & The Frequent Meal Myth

I have done my best workouts during a fasted state. Besides feeling really good during working out in a fasted state, training this way is the best way I have personally found to stay lean.

Does everybody have to train fasted? No, of course not; people are all different. If you feel good training in a fasted state, you can train ideally just before you break your fast. Once you are finished training, jump on the first meal of the day. Something proponents of intermittent fasting are also suggesting nowadays is having a whey protein shake before your workout. This can be done without considering it as breaking your fast and theoretically, it can help with your muscle building goals. I have been doing this the last couple of months, but I haven't really seen any differences in my physique or workout productivity. Keep in mind that I achieved all of my big results in physique and strength without any supplements; so don't worry if having a protein shake before your workout is not an option.

Important note: Make sure you have a fulfilling meal rich in carbs and protein the day before you train in a fasted state.

4

How clean should your diet be?

Yes, CLEAN EATING can help most of you (including me) stay lean or even lose weight. Well, in the short run at least. It's common for people to end up harming their health by eating strictly clean because they think that they can have as much "clean" calories as they want. Clean eating allows you to have whole and minimally processed foods such as rice, vegetables, chicken, etc. and restricts, or even eliminates, items such as sweets and "junk" food from your diet. Clean foods play an important part of a healthy diet due to their nutritional value and the satiety they provide. However, making them the only food choices allowed, becomes not only boring but eventually also repressive. As Anthony de Mello once said:

> *"Every time you renounce something,*
> *you are eternally tied to it"*

Try the following experiment. Think of a food category you don't mind eating but you are also not crazy about. For me that would be something like legumes. Now imagine that someone told you, you could never have this food again. Imagine this scenario very vividly for a couple of minutes and you will probably end salivating over a food you thought you never really cared about (I'm craving brown beans this moment). Now imagine what happens once you renounce majestic foods such as ice-cream. Besides the fact that you'll be constantly obsessing over ice-cream, there will come a day when you will just end up binging on it and probably get back most of the calories you skipped.

How Clean Should Your Diet Be?
Enter Flexible Dieting

Especially once you reach a weight you are happy with, the key to sustaining it long-term is a diet that can be flexible. What is most important is that a diet should suit your lifestyle and cover your personal needs in nutrients and calories. Avoid extreme diets that completely exclude food categories. For example, there is no concrete scientific evidence that excluding meat from your diet by going vegetarian is a healthier choice. Sure eating too much meat might be bad, but even water in excess can be harmful for your health. If you are not exceeding your calories and if you are covering your needs in macronutrients (proteins, fats, carbs) and micronutrients (vitamins & minerals) you can have some of the "dirty" stuff. Here are some basic guidelines for a healthy & flexible diet:

<u>1. Eat primarily real and minimally processed food.</u>

Prefer products that are the end result of sun, air, water and earth. In other words, you should be able to kill it, grow it out of the earth or pick it off a tree.

This doesn't mean that you can't have some junk food or sweets every now and then. Keeping a diet that consists 80-90% of healthy and minimally processed food is the key to a balanced diet and maintaining a healthy eating behavior. Diets that completely exclude foods only lead to huge binge eating episodes and other unhealthy eating behaviors in the long run. For example, if most of your calorie intake was from healthy foods today, it's ok to have something sweet or a small portion of junk food meal at the end of the day. Just try to keep it around 200-300 calories. If you ate clean the whole week, it's ok to have a bigger indulgence on the weekend.

Personally, I prefer keeping it 95% "clean" during the week and inside my house. I avoid having junk lying around the kitchen. Even if I'm not hungry, I know that if I see those oreos lying around it will be difficult to resist. On the weekend I eat around 75% clean. I allow myself more of the fun stuff so that when I go out with friends or have social commitments, I don't end up being the weird guy who says I'm on a diet while the rest of the group is having beer, eating pizza and having fun. Either you want it or not, if you're a clean eater you will eventually become an outsider in such situations. If I happen to go out on a Thursday night I switch that day with my weekend day.

2. Eat Enough Calories According To Your Own Needs.

Someone who spends his whole day working in an office does not have the same caloric needs as a construction worker. Calculate how many calories your body needs and have a basic awareness of the amount of caloric content the foods you eat on a daily basis.

3. Have Protein With Every Meal.

Protein is the most satiating macronutrient and together with healthy fats they are the two most essential macronutrients for health. You could survive without carbs in your diet for example, but not without protein and fat. Every year more and more scientific studies report the importance of a protein rich diet for appetite control and weight loss. It is also as we all know an essential macronutrient for building muscle. Try to include at least a bit of protein in all of your meals. Examples: Have some nuts with your fruits, have some Feta cheese with your salad or have an omelet in the morning rather than a sugary bowl of cereal.

4. Eat Slower

Slow eating can aid digestion and give you a more long-lasting satisfaction from every meal. This will help you eat less on a daily basis.

Flexible Dieting is Practical But Not Easy

I see a tendency among former clean eaters to go to the other end of the spectrum once they get off the clean eating wagon. It's easy to misunderstand flexible dieting and think that there is no effort required to follow a healthy flexible diet. The truth is that flexible dieting may allow you a bit of all the yummy stuff but that doesn't make it easy. You still need to put some effort into it, to be organized, and constantly work on healthy eating habits. After all, if eating healthy and being ripped was easy, everyone would be doing it.

5

My secret weight-loss strategy

IF YOU WANT to lose a large amount of weight, then you might have to modify IF a little bit after a certain point. IF works great if you are doing it for the first time, but after a certain point you might hit a weight loss plateau. Begin with regular IF and once you reach that plateau start abstaining from carbs during the day until you have your main meal at dinner. During the day, eat vegetables, fruits and food with healthy fats and rich in protein like meat, eggs, yogurts, kefir, cottage cheese, etc. Go for easily digestive meat sources, such as fish and poultry. A similar approach is used in Ori Hofmekler's - Warrior diet, and I see it as a helpful progression of intermittent fasting once you reach a weight plateau.

At the end of the day, enjoy yourself with a fulfilling meal rich in vegetables, carbs and protein. If some of you are thinking that eating a bit meal late at night might make you gain weight, that's also another outdated myth drawn as a faulty conclusion from epidemiological studies in the past. If you eat a lot during the day and then eat again a lot during the evening, guess what? You will gain weight, of course! It's simple calorie math. But if you control your calorie intake during the day so that you have more room for extra calories during the evening hours, this problem will not occur.

Knowing that you will end your day with a satisfying dinner will make it a lot easier to stay disciplined during the rest of the day. After a long day, once you're done with all your busy responsibilities you are in the perfect relaxed state to properly eat and digest a nice, warm and fulfilling meal. Enjoy – you earned it!

<u>Helpfull tips to avoid overeating during your last main meal of the day:</u>

1. **Start your meal with vegetables**. Get the healthy stuff out of the way otherwise it's easy to fill yourself up with rice and steak and end up skipping your salad. Filling yourself up with some veggies in the beginning of the meal will help you reach satiety faster.
2. **After your veggies, continue with your carbs and protein.**
3. **Eat slow and be aware of the process.** Enjoy every bite of your meal and learn to eat consciously. It's very important for reaching satiety faster. Avoid things like eating in front of the TV.
4. **Have a glass of water on the table.** Drinking some water together with your meal can also help with satiety. Don't overdo it though because more than a glass can disrupt digestion for some people.

5. **Have dessert only when it's worth it.** You can have a little piece of your favorite dessert now and then. If your favorite dessert is on the table don't torture yourself to avoid eating it. This can and in most cases does lead to binge eating later on. However, don't eat dessert just because it happens to be around. Learn to apply some discipline, when it's do-able.

6. **Tip to avoid overeating - brush your teeth.** Sometimes no matter what we do, even if we feel we've had enough, we have an uncontrollable feeling of greedy hunger that wants us to keep on going. A cool trick to avoid this from happening is during your last meal of the day, brush your teeth once you feel you've had enough. Most people don't feel like eating after their mouth is clean and fresh, especially since it makes many foods taste bad. If brushing your teeth isn't practical at the moment, a good mouthwash can also work.

Helpfull tips to avoid overeating during the rest of the day:

1. **Stay Busy.** The best way not to over eat is not to have too much free time to think about eating in the first place. The best way I have found to avoid eating too much is to stay busy, doing stuff I enjoy. Arrange daily tasks during the times of the day when hunger strikes when you usually want to indulge in all kinds of calorie dense temptations.

2. **Walk.** If you have a sedentary lifestyle, if your work doesn't require any physical activity, you need to add some extra

movement in your life. My choice of movement is walking. I just put a good audiobook in my mp3 and go walk for an hour, at least 3 times a week. Find a nice calm place to walk, it will also help clear your mind, it can improve your sleep if you do it in the evening and its also a great way to start your morning. Regardless of where or when, what is most important is that you plan time in your schedule to get some movement. If you don't like walking, an alternative is to jog for 30-40 minutes instead, play some football or basketball with your friends, swim, ski, play with your kids, whatever physical activity you prefer, just find a way to include movement in your daily schedule. Skip the elevator, don't take the car/bicycle/motorbike. Do it the old fashion way - use your legs!

Important note: The fact that you add some movement in your life is not an excuse to eat more. Walk to feed your body with movement not to feed your body with calories afterwards.

Training on a fasted state
If you have a good fulfilling meal before you start fasting; you can last a lot more than 16 hours on a fasted state in order for your liver's glycogen stores to run out and begin the muscle breakdown to re-fuel you. If you want to be 100% sure that you're on the safe side, I would not recommend prolonging your fasts the days you train for more than 16 hours. The only thing your muscles may lose during a fast is muscle glycogen (sugar) which will be replenished after you have a meal rich in carbohydrates.

6

The truth about supplements

ALMOST ALL SUPPLEMENTS promise extreme results, by misleading and brainwashing many people in the exercise-fitness community. In my experience, if your diet and our lifestyle are perfect, supplements will may offer your muscle building goals an extra 5% help (and half of that might just be a placebo effect). Just to be clear, I am not anti-supplement. I just find it too boring to deal with most supplements in my daily schedule because I just prefer eating and spending money on real food.

Supplements supported by Science:

1. Protein Supplements. Increased protein consumption has been proven to aid athletic muscle building goals. Do you need protein powder for this? The answer is no. You can get all your protein through your diet if you want and it makes no difference if you take no protein supplements. The reason protein supplements are helpful is because they are practical. Not everybody can eat a ton of meat and other protein rich food sources on a daily basis. We have busy schedules, we don't always have the luxury of cooking our meals and finding proper sources of protein when eating outside is not always possible (and for a lot of us it's also very costly). Quality meat in the Netherlands for example (which is were I'm residing at the moment) is quite expensive. A scoop of quality protein costs less than 1 euro when at the same time getting the same grams of quality protein can cost me quadruple that price. I don't mean you should substitute dietary protein with powder protein. If you can afford it, by all means get all the quality protein you can. Fill your fridge with salmon, eggs, beef and all of that good stuff.

Some people are afraid that protein supplements can cause kidney problems. The only category of people that might be in danger by a very high protein diet are people with kidney issues and this category of people is often used as a faulty generalization by mass media or other people to criticize high protein diets. Yes, protein requires more effort by your kidneys to be processed, but guess what? The kidneys are always under stress! That's what they're made for. About 20% of the blood pumped by the heart goes to the kidneys and they filter a total of 180 liters (48 gallons) of blood every single day.

Adding some more protein to your diet may increase their workload a little, but it is really insignificant compared to the immense amount of work that they do already. A study examining bodybuilders with protein intakes of 2.8g/kg vs. well-trained athletes with moderate protein intakes revealed no significant differences in kidney function between the groups. Additionally, a review of the scientific literature on protein intake and renal function concluded that "there is no reason to restrict protein in healthy individuals."

Personally, I keep a protein whey supplement around the house and use it mostly in the following scenarios:

a) On days that I skip a meal due to being too busy;
b) When I can't afford foods like a big juicy grass fed steak to cover my high protein needs; or
c) When I feel like having a pre-workout liquid meal after fasting intermitted.

2. Creatine Monohydrate has been shown to improve power output and is often used by athletes to increase high-intensity exercise capacity and lean body mass. It is one of the most studied supplements and it has been proven to aid muscle building goals very effectively. Most Studies show that supplementing with creatine properly doesn't cause health issues as some people fear. Keep in mind, however, that there are a fair amount of people who are non-responders, so there is a possibility that you won't see any results by adding this supplement. I don't have a lot to say on this topic since I don't have enough personal experience with this supplement to offer you any anecdotal insight.

3. **Beta-alanine** is a modified version of the amino acid alanine and it has been shown to enhance muscular endurance. Many people report being able to perform one or two additional reps in the gym when training in sets of 8-15 repetitions and it's a supplement often combined with Creatine. Once again, I don't have any

personal experience with this supplement to offer you any anecdotal insight.

My Secret Supplement

Oh, this is another substance I forgot to mention that also has been proven to be effective. I use a caffeine supplement as a pre and intra-workout supplement most of the days I train. It's inexpensive, you can easily find it at the supermarket and it's called - Coffee! You add a teaspoon of it in water, stir and drink. I prefer ice coffee during the warm months of the year and hot coffee when it's cold. I do this regardless if I'm training fasted or not. Having a cup of coffee is more of a ritual than a pre-workout for me. I love sipping some hot or ice coffee while I'm preparing my training music list and checking my notes in my training log from the previous workout.

Doesn't Coffee Dehydrate You?

Someone recently asked me if coffee is ok as a pre and intra-workout drink during intermittent fasting because it is said to dehydrate the body. This is just another myth, coffee just as any drink can contribute to your daily fluid requirement. Coffee as part of a normal lifestyle doesn't cause fluid loss in excess of the volume ingested. Yes it does have a mild diuretic effect but it doesn't appear to increase the risk of dehydration. Of course anything in excess is not good for you (not even plain water) so avoid extreme coffee consumption. Here is how I deal with my coffee "addiction." Because I love the taste of coffee and enjoy drink it often during the day, I have small cups (1/2 of normal cup) and drink it light and plain (no sugar or milk). This way I drink about 5-6 cups a day but its more like 2-3 cups

P.S. Sometimes in the afternoon I splurge and add some milk and sugar in my last cup!

Final thoughts on supplements

As you can see my experience with supplements is quite limited but I considered it important to mention them since this is an important topic that many people frequently ask questions about. The three supplements above are the only a few that are backed up by serious scientific research and are the only few proven to work. If you want to supplement your athletic diet it's up to you. Make sure you choose a quality manufacturer and just to be on the safe side ask a nutritionist for some extra guidelines referring to dosage and any implications they might have with your other dietary habits and/or medications.

My advice is to find the weak links in your lifestyle and diet and if you cannot fix them naturally, ask a specialist for advice on how to address these needs. Don't forget however, supplements are not magical and won't give you any significant results, especially if you don't train hard enough. As a matter of fact, a poor diet with a good training program will give you greater results than an average training program combined with the perfect diet and the finest powder and pill supplements.

Don't obsess over supplements. I find that a lot of people spend too much time worrying over supplements which distracts them from what really delivers results - Hard work.

7

Final thoughts on Nutrition

ONE OF THE most essential characteristics of a diet is that it should be sustainable in the long run. The word diet originates from the Greek word Dieta (δίαιτα) and it relates to dieting as a way of living. If you keep on hopping from one diet to another and one binge episode to another after each time you try to eat healthy, you are simply moving one step forward and two steps backwards. There is no progress and you are creating unhealthy eating behaviors. The only way that you will able to control your weight long term is if you turn your diet into a long lasting lifestyle that vitalizes you, keeps your mind clear, keeps you healthy, doesn't make you over-weight and as a result of all the above makes you happy.

The environment we live in today, as well as the way we are wired through evolution in order to survive, make us easily prone to obesity. However, we are also equipped with the capabilities of forming new habits, developing awareness of our actions and cultivating discipline. It might be easier to blame nutritional myths for the reason why people become obese but the truth is as simple as basic principles of thermodynamics. If you consume more caloric-fuel than the energy you produce, you will gain weight. Be a grown up and learn to take responsibility. Admit that if you're not satisfied with your weight it's because you prefer sitting rather than moving. Finding pleasure in overeating is a bigger priority to you than health and self-confidence. This also goes for the skinny guys who complain about not being able to gain weight. If you want to gain weight, stop complaining about how hard it is and organize your calorie intake. Plan more frequent and bigger meals and do more strength training. You need to take action, period.

Start With The Basics.
Don't start strict diets before you begin with the basics. What are the basics? Start doing what your mother told you when you were young...

1. **Eat all your vegetables.** Eat at least three portions a day, I like to eat a huge veggie mix before dinner.
2. **Eat fruits.** Try to eat at least two portions a day.
3. **Eat all your food.** Eat the appropriate amount of calories your body needs

Now go clean up your room...

Start with these basic guidelines and you'll be eating healthier than 80% of the people out there. Doing extreme/express diets every year for a couple of weeks to lose weight rapidly only puts stress on your body and mind and usually leads to regaining the weight you lost. Constantly seeking instant pleasure in junk food may make you feel better temporary but always has a larger negative impact on your physical and mental health in the long-run. If you understand all the above, then you will know that putting in the effort to create a proper and organized diet on a weekly basis is the smart thing to do.

*"To eat is a necessity, but to eat
intelligently is an art"*

- La Rochefoucauld

Final thoughts on Homemade Muscle

MOST PEOPLE WANT an aesthetic physique. Wanting though is very different from willing to do what is required to achieve this goal. They fail because they always find excuses along the way. When I was developing this home workout program, I had a severely fractured leg, which means I had to train most of the time with full leg casts, special fracture boots and crutches. Of course, I don't advise people recovering from bone fractures to train hardcore using bodyweight exercises. My point here is that if you want to get into shape, you have to stop finding excuses.

Socrates, the ancient Greek philosopher said, "It is a disgrace for someone to grow old without ever seeing the beauty and strength of which your body is capable." Time flies by us faster than we realize and one day it will be too late to make a difference. So stop disrespecting your body, get off the couch and start strengthening body and mind! There is only one thing that can get between you and your aspirations, and that is you!

*"It is a disgrace for someone to grow old without
ever seeing the beauty and strength of
which his body is capable"*

Common Excuses Your Mind Will Use Against You to Avoid Working Out

1) Limited Time

On average, this program takes 3 hours per week of your time. A week has 168 hours, so training 3 hours per week means you have to spend less than 2% of your week in order to accomplish your goals. Anybody can sacrifice that amount of time in order to get in shape and to look and feel better.

2) Fear of Failure

Sometimes we just make up excuses to avoid chasing our goals, because we are afraid. This fear may be conscious or subconscious but it's there...it's the fear of failure. We are too scared that we might put time and effort into something that has no guarantee of success. A lot of us fail in our minds before we even start. Fear is nothing we should run away from though. Fear is a natural human emotion and there is no need to consider it a negative one. On the contrary, it means you are getting out of your comfort zone, which is the only place you can find place for growth. When fear shows up at your door, say hello and invite it in; become friends with it. The more you push it away, the more it insists on re-visiting.

Accept your fears but don't be a coward...

3) Laziness

Sloth (laziness) is another great enemy everyone faces when they set a goal, especially when it comes to exercise. We make excuses to cover our indolence because we are simply too attached to immediate gratification in favor of long-term growth. Evolutionarily it makes sense to always go for the sure bet - to eat that candy in front of us right now. Our ancestors didn't have to worry about becoming overweight or heart disease. Our brain evolved in a world where we probably wouldn't live long enough to meet your grandchildren. The primitive part of our brain wants us to gobble up anything edible around us and reserve as much energy possible. In simple words, it wants us to strive to be fat and lazy!

How to train when life gets in the way

Your training program won't always run as smoothly as shown in training tables of exercise books. There will be periods when life will just happen. Unexpected events will get in your way. You or other people will get sick and life in general will be tough. Keep in mind that I don't expect you to always consider these events the easy way out. I have days when I have leg problems, when I sleep less, or train at different times (which I hate because I'm a control freak). Some days I have to force myself to get through the workout because I know that after completing it I will feel better.

The 90-20 Axiom: Anytime you feel like not working out remember this self-evident truth: 90% of the times you feel physically or mentally tired it's only the first 20% of the workout that you will have to push yourself through. Once you get past the warm-up and maybe a couple of sets into your workout, you will get into it and you will be happy you got started after all.

Missing your passion for exercise

Still, even if you develop a passionate relationship with exercise, there will always be periods in your life when you won't want to exercise at all. As with any long-term relationship, passion always comes and goes through time. During difficult periods, when you feel you have no flame in your heart for working out, it is quite easy to just let go and see all your hard work disappear. Less than forty days for most people is enough time to see more than half of their results disappear. When we experience this lack of passion, it's important to avoid the following two mistakes:

1. Pushing it too hard. When you're going through a rough patch and you have no desire at all to workout, if you push yourself to train as hard as you always do, you will usually end up resenting your workout.

2. Quitting entirely. When there is no inner motivation to exercise it's also easy to completely quit on your workouts. This usually happens when you are having too much fun doing other stuff or because you are too depressed to do anything at all. The end result is that you end up dismissing your fitness goals all at once.

If you're going through such periods, learn to train just enough to maintain your current condition. Don't think about progress, breaking plateaus and don't worry if you come short a couple of reps from your usual routine. Just shut your brain off and do a couple of sets for the basic three movement patterns. Pull, Push and Squat. The following training plan contains two fifteen minute training sessions that will keep you in shape during such times. Even at our darkest hours, we can all find time and energy to work out 30 minutes a week.

	Exercises	Sets	Reps	Rest between sets	Rest between exercises
Multijoint exercises	1. Pull-ups	3			
	3. Pistol Squats	3	5 -15	1 MINUTE	2 MINUTES
	4. Handstand Push-ups	3			

Do this two times per week...

*"You don't develop courage by being happy in
your relationships every day. You develop it by
surviving difficult times and challenging adversity"*

~ Epicurus

Weights or Bodyweight Exercise - What is Better?

Exercise benefits both body and mind. Studies have shown that aerobic and strength training can help battle feelings of depression. The antidepressant effect of exercise has been shown in studies to be just as effective as that of antidepressant drugs. In general, the more you include healthy movement in your lifestyle the better your chances are to feel better. If you have major depression related issues, I am not suggesting you should quit taking the medication your doctor might have prescribed for you. I am simply recommending adding some exercise on top of that and see what happens.

Even if you reach a point in life when physical growth will stop, when there will be no more space for building stronger muscle fibers or improving your neuromuscular coordination, that momentum you've gained from physical growth through strength training will keep you growing internally.

Homemade Muscle is not against training at the gym or any other kind of strength exercise. Homemade Muscle is about motivating you to be strong no matter what your circumstances are. Still I have to give you my opinion. I have to tell you, which out of the two I consider superior. I started these workouts because they were the only alternative I had at the moment. Nowadays if I had to choose between working out at the gym or using bodyweight exercise, without a blink of an eye, my answer would be bodyweight exercise. It still remains the only form of exercise I do.

<u>I don't care what others say:</u>

- No gym pushing exercise can beat handstand push-ups
- No gym pulling machine can beat pull-ups
- No gym crunching machine can beat dragon flags
- No gym machine and beat one-arm push ups.

If you want to get the most out of both worlds, my suggestion would be adding barbell squats to the lower body exercises of this program while using weighted lunges as warm-up sets (that is, once you're strong enough to perform them). Maybe I'll write a program like that in the future. As I said previously, if having to choose between the two, bodyweight exercise is the best and ultimate form of strength exercise in my opinion.

Here are the basic reasons I know this to be true:

1) Reward: Gaining greater self-mastery and control of your own body by conquering new bodyweight progressions and skills is one of the most functional, empowering, motivational and rewarding feelings exercise can provide.

2) Symmetry: Bodyweight exercise develops balanced strength and builds the body as a whole. There is no room for a weak core when you are doing exercises like handstand push-ups. The moment you lose connection between your upper and lower body through a weak core, you will start shaking like a leaf.

3) Ultimate Self-Mastery: The feeling of self-mastery you attain by mastering your physical self also carries over to self-mastery of your inner world. Balance your body and you will find balance in life. Strengthen your muscles and your mind will follow. The reward that comes after patience and persistence develops a mindset that can help you deal with most of life's other challenges.

"Mastering Bodyweight Exercises trumps
working out at the Gym"

~ Homemade Muscle

Exercise Menu

Developing the Zen mindset

PEOPLE HAVE TOLD me that exercises, such as the one-arm pull ups, are only for those born strong. This always made my goals a bit intimidating, but there's nothing I love more than proving people wrong. I was never the strongest guy of the group. I also never was the underdog of my sports teams. But, I also never believed genetics can define you to a great extent. One of the most important mindsets you have to develop in life is to never let someone's opinion of you become your reality. I got my first one arm pull-up after two years of serious bodyweight training because I never let people around me set my limitations. One arm push-ups, dragon flags, and even one arm pull-ups can be achieved if you continue to focus on steady and gradual progress.

Pick progressions in every exercise that are suitable for you and just keep on hammering them. You have to develop a Zen mindset..

"Stay thirsty but do not become impatient. Let
there be emotional yearning but avoid frustration.

If you obsess about it, it will never happen.
Just like a seed doesn't seem to be blossoming into
a flower if you keep on staring at it... Be patient
and it will come naturally, on its own terms".

Exercises, like handstand push-ups, might sound too tough for you if you're a beginner. However, remember that your goal is to work yourself up through easier progressions. Personally, it took me 5 months to get 5 clean reps of handstand push-ups! On the other hand, I've seen people do them within two weeks of training. Today, handstand push-ups are one of my top three favorite exercises for strength training. If you would tell me you only have time for three exercises, I would tell you to pick Handstand push-ups, Pull-ups and weighted lunges.

"Don't let someone else's opinion of you
become your reality".

~ Les Brown

Recommended Equipment (optional)

Full disclosure -- I have no connection with the
company that makes these items.

As you will see below in the exercise tutorial, I offer ways to do each exercise without any equipment. Still, I believe a Pull-up bar is a must if you want this workout plan to be efficient. I personally use the Iron Gym pull-up bar which currently costs around 30 dollars. It has three grip positions, narrow, wide, and neutral which come in handy. It uses leverage to hold against the doorway, so there are no screws and no need to damage your door. Plus it's quite easy to assemble. If you visit their website you can easily find a local retailer in your neighborhood.

After that, if you want to invest some more money on bodyweight equipment, I would also recommend a dip station. The main reason I recommend a dip station is that it's friendlier for your wrists. The one I use is called "Ultimate Body Press Dip Stand." For its value, it's the best dip stand I have found around the web and currently costs about 90 dollars. It is a simple piece of equipment made of steel construction that snaps together. It's ideal for dips and inverted rows. You can easily pack it and transport it in a car and It goes together and comes apart in seconds. The only problem you might have with it is if you are on the tall side; so check the dimensions at the manufacturer's website if you decide to purchase it.

Video Tutorials

If a picture is worth a thousand words then one could say that a video is worth a thousand images. When it comes to demonstrating an exercise I'm not a fan of merely using text and images as in most books. I believe that it's essential for the trainer to demonstrate an exercise live, but since I can't train every single reader of this book (although I'd love to) I have made a page with video tutorials from my YouTube channel for every single exercise. You can also find other helpful stuff such as "How to make a homemade weighted back pack" etc...

Just visit: **www.homemademuscle.com/tutorials**

A lot of these are the first videos I made once I got back on my feet (or foot to be accurate), after my accident. I hope you can withstand lack of experience with cameras, my lame presentation skills and my once introverted awkwardness! Still the technique and demonstration are solid so move pass all the above and focus on form!

END NOTES

Doing an exercise with good form, contrary to doing an exercise with bad form, can play a huge role on the difficulty of it, and injury prevention. Just the feeling that you are performing an exercise correctly, doesn't always mean you actually are. It's important to pay close attention and observe your form. You can use mirrors, or ask someone experienced to spot you while exercising. Almost every cell phone has a camera today, so you can also use your phone or any other device available for you, and film your trainings to see how your form looks. If you notice mistakes, write them down and focus on them next time.

Having the perfect technique in every single rep and every single moment is not always possible, not even by professionals. But that doesn't mean you shouldn't try. As one of my favorite quotes says,

"Perfection is not attainable, but if we chase perfection we can catch excellence"

~ Vince Lombardi

BEFORE YOU GO 3 THINGS...

1) Motivation

As a popular quote by Zig Ziglar says

"People often say that motivation doesn't last. Well, neither does bathing, that's why we recommend it daily."

So how do you get motivated on a daily basis? Start by finding people that inspire you and surround yourself with them. Thanks to the internet and social media you can find these kind of people with a click of a button. Like pages that support your goals and follow people who have accomplished what you're aiming for. For example, if you liked this book then make sure you like my Facebook page and follow me on Instagram.

Here is what you'll see on my Facebook page at facebook.com/HomeMadeMuscles

- Motivational videos and photos
- Nutritional tips
- Exercise tips
- Video Tutorials (exercises, workouts, recipes)
- Articles (exercise, workouts, nutrition)

Follow me on Instagram page www.Instagram.com/Homemade Muscles

- Food pictures (get ideas on what to cook and healthy muscle building food)
- Motivational quotes
- Motivational exercise videos and photos

Subscribe to my Youtube Channel:.Youtube.com/user/Home MadeMuscles/

- Daily Nutritional tips
- Daily Exercise tips
- Tutorials (exercises, workouts, recipes)
- Meditation tips
- Free ebooks (I always share 99% of my books for free the first 3 days I release them!)

2) Action

As we said motivation is required but it's not enough on it's own. None of all this matters unless you start taking action... No matter how many exercise, diet and self-development books you read - nothing changes without self-practice. Make sure you're theoretical practice doesn't outweigh your actual/physical practice.

"Knowing is not enough, you must apply; willing is not enough, you must do"

~Bruce Lee

Did this book add value to your life?

Support my project by leaving me a review!

(A few honest words from the heart are enough..)

Made in the USA
Lexington, KY
20 March 2016